Sexual Dysfunction in Men and Women

Edited by

Stanley Zaslau, MD, MBA, FACS
Professor
Urology Residency Program Director
Division of Urology
West Virginia University
Morgantown, West Virginia

LIBRARY

College of Physicians and Surgeons
of British Columbia

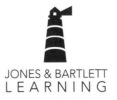

JONES & BARTLETT
LEARNING

LIBRARY - CPSBC

000000MLS49547

World Headquarters

Jones & Bartlett Learning
40 Tall Pine Drive
Sudbury, MA 01776
978-443-5000
info@jblearning.com
www.jblearning.com

Jones & Bartlett Learning Canada
6339 Ormindale Way
Mississauga, Ontario L5V 1J2
Canada

Jones & Bartlett Learning International
Barb House, Barb Mews
London W6 7PA
United Kingdom

Jones & Bartlett Learning books and products are available through most bookstores and
online booksellers. To contact Jones & Bartlett Learning directly, call 800-832-0034,
fax 978-443-8000, or visit our website, www.jblearning.com.

Substantial discounts on bulk quantities of Jones & Bartlett Learning publications are
available to corporations, professional associations, and other qualified organizations.
For details and specific discount information, contact the special sales department
at Jones & Bartlett Learning via the above contact information or send an email to
specialsales@jblearning.com.

Copyright © 2011 by Jones & Bartlett Learning, LLC

All rights reserved. No part of the material protected by this copyright may be reproduced
or utilized in any form, electronic or mechanical, including photocopying, recording, or
by any information storage and retrieval system, without written permission from the
copyright owner.

The authors, editor, and publisher have made every effort to provide accurate information.
However, they are not responsible for errors, omissions, or for any outcomes related to the
use of the contents of this book and take no responsibility for the use of the products
and procedures described. Treatments and side effects described in this book may not be
applicable to all people; likewise, some people may require a dose or experience a side
effect that is not described herein. Drugs and medical devices are discussed that may have
limited availability controlled by the Food and Drug Administration (FDA) for use only in a
research study or clinical trial. Research, clinical practice, and government regulations often
change the accepted standard in this field. When consideration is being given to use of any
drug in the clinical setting, the healthcare provider or reader is responsible for determining
FDA status of the drug, reading the package insert, and reviewing prescribing information
for the most up-to-date recommendations on dose, precautions, and contraindications, and
determining the appropriate usage for the product. This is especially important in the case
of drugs that are new or seldom used.

Production Credits

Executive Publisher: Christopher Davis
Production Director: Amy Rose
Senior Acquisitions Editor: Nancy Anastasi Duffy
Editorial Assistant: Sara Cameron
Senior Production Editor: Daniel Stone
Associate Production Editor: Jill Morton
Associate Marketing Manager: Katie Hennessy
V.P., Manufacturing and Inventory Control: Therese
Connell
Composition: Dedicated Business
Solutions
Cover Design: Kate Ternullo
Cover Image: © Anna Marynenko/
ShutterStock, Inc.
Printing and Binding: Malloy
Incorporated
Cover Printing: Malloy Incorporated

Library of Congress Cataloging-in-Publication Data
Dx/Rx : sexual dysfunction in men and women / edited by Stanley Zaslau.
    p. ; cm.
  Includes bibliographical references and index.
  ISBN-13: 978-0-7637-7196-6
  ISBN-10: 0-7637-7196-1
  1. Sexual disorders—Handbooks, manuals, etc. I. Zaslau, Stanley. II. Title: Sexual
dysfunction in men and women.
  [DNLM: 1. Sexual Dysfunction, Physiological. 2. Female Urogenital Diseases—
therapy. 3. Male Urogenital Diseases—therapy. WJ 709 D993 2012]
  RC556.D95 2012
  616.85'83—dc22
                                                      2010025508
6048

Printed in the United States of America
14 13 12 11 10   10 9 8 7 6 5 4 3 2 1

Dedication

To our urology residents, past, present, and future, whose interest in and enthusiasm for enhancing their knowledge invigorate us to continue our role as educators.

Contents

Editor's Preface

It is our belief that sexual dysfunction is a common condition affecting both men and women. Many practitioners, particularly in the disciplines of family practice, internal medicine, and urology, may have the opportunity to treat both male and female patients, sometimes even the husband and wife of a family. In such instances, sexual dysfunction may be occurring in both partners. For that reason, we decided to present information regarding the pathogenesis, diagnosis, and treatment of sexual dysfunction in men and women in the same book. The book is well supplemented with tables and timely references. Any practitioner who deals with both male and female patients with sexual problems will find this book to be useful.

Stanley Zaslau
Morgantown, West Virginia

Contributors

■ Editor

Stanley Zaslau, MD, MBA, FACS
Professor
Urology Residency Program Director
Division of Urology
West Virginia University
Morgantown, West Virginia

■ Contributing Authors

Aimee Rogers, MD
Senior Resident
Division of Urology
West Virginia University
Morgantown, West Virginia

Adam Luchey, MD
Senior Resident
Division of Urology
West Virginia University
Morgantown, West Virginia

Chad P. Hubscher, MD
Resident
Division of Urology
West Virginia University
Morgantown, West Virginia

Male Sexual Dysfunction

CHAPTER 1

Physiology of Erection

Aimee Rogers, MD ■ *Stanley Zaslau, MD, MBA, FACS*

■ Introduction

- Penile erection is the result of increased penile inflow of blood and reduced outflow.
  - Arterial inflow of blood to the penis is coupled with vasodilation of the cavernosal and helicine arteries.
  - This results in blood filling the sinusoidal spaces of the corpora cavernosa.
  - This leads to expansion of the lacunar spaces and tunica albuginea.
- Neural control of erection involves a shift from sympathetic tone to parasympathetic tone.
- The neural circuitry for erection is based in the spinal cord.

■ Role of Spinal Cord and Neural Innervation of the Penis

- The penis receives autonomic innervation from the sympathetic and parasympathetic nervous systems.
- Both systems contain nuclei located in the spinal cord.
- The parasympathetic nervous system is excitatory for erectile function.
  - Preganglionic parasympathetic neurons arise from the sacral spinal cord segments S2–S4.
  - The major segment contributing to erectile function is S3.
- The sympathetic nervous system is inhibitory to erectile function.
  - However, because of its vasoconstrictive properties, some fibers have a role in pelvic vasoconstriction, which may increase blood flow to the penis to promote erection.

- The nuclei for the sympathetic nervous system are located in the intermediolateral cell column and the dorsal gray horn at the thoracolumbar cord.
- Preganglionic sympathetic fibers arise from T11–L2 segments of the spinal cord.
- The dorsal nerve of the penis contains the sensory afferents from the penis.

■ Most penile erections occur as a result of the complex interplay of the peripheral and central nervous systems in an intact spinal cord, as described above. However, penile erections can also occur as a result of local stimulation.

■ Hormonal Control of Sexuality

■ There are a wide variety of hormones that play a role in control and potentiation of sexuality.

■ Much of the knowledge of these hormones has been achieved through the study of animal models.

■ **Table 1.1** lists these important hormones that control sexuality. The role of each of these hormones and their contribution to sexuality will be described in detail following the table.

Serotonin

■ There are a large number of serotonin (5-HT) positive neurons in the central nervous system.

■ 5-HT is felt to have an overall inhibitory effect on male sexual functions.

- Johnson and colleagues found that stimulation of the 5-HT nuclei of the spinal cord diminishes the responsiveness of the dorsal nerve of the penis.[1]

Table 1.1 Important Hormones in the Control of Sexuality

Serotonin
Norepinephrine
Dopamine
Nitric oxide
Oxytocin
Adrenocorticotropic hormone
Melanocyte-stimulating hormone

- Several 5-HT receptors have been identified and have been divided into classes.
  - The 5-HT1A receptor is thought to facilitate sexual behavior.
  - The 5-HT1B receptor is thought to inhibit ejaculatory behavior.
    - In a rat study by Ahlenius and colleagues, the increased ejaculatory latency produced by 5-HTP was blocked by treatment with isamoltane, a 5-HT1B receptor antagonist.[2]
    - This group also studied the selective serotonin reuptake inhibitor citalopram and found that it did not affect the male rat ejaculatory behavior.

Norepinephrine

- There is anatomical suggestion of the importance of adrenergic control in the physiology of erection.
  - Yaici and associates have shown that sympathetic and parasympathetic preganglionic neurons that innervate the penis are adjacent to the neural endpoints for the alpha 2 a and c adrenoreceptor subtypes.[3]
  - Kaplan and colleagues have shown that epinephrine can inhibit erectile activity through its actions on alpha 1 adrenoreceptors.[4]
- The location of adrenergic control of sexual behavior may be central as well as peripheral.
  - Morales and associates have shown that yohimbine, a centrally acting alpha 2 antagonist, can stimulate sexual motivation in male rats.[5]
  - However, Ernst and associates, through systematic review and meta-analysis of randomized clinical trials, have shown limited clinical efficacy of yohimbine versus placebo in human subjects.[6]

Dopamine

- Dopamine's prosexual effect was noticed through the observation that Parkinson's patients treated with dopamine agonists had increased sexual activity.
  - Uitti and colleagues identified 13 parkinsonian patients who experienced hypersexuality as a consequence of

anti-parkinsonian therapy.[7] The majority of patients were men and had a relatively early onset of Parkinson's symptoms. There was no relation between functional Parkinson's improvement and increased sexuality.

- In rats, apomorphine is a proerectogenic agent. However, in humans, it appears to have a facilitatory effect. Thus, its likelihood of improving erectile function is minimal.

- Dopamine may exert its possible role in erectile function through several structures, such as:
  - The nucleus accumbens
    - May or may not have a significant role in dopamine's function of sexuality. Results with study of rats have been contradictory to date.
  - The medial preoptic area
    - This area appears to have prosexual effects.
  - The paraventricular nucleus of the hypothalamus
    - According to a study by Melis and colleagues, this area can respond to injection doses of apomorphine and induce erections in rats.[8]
    - In this study, both penile erection and yawning behavior were noted.
      - This secondary effect of apomorphine has limited this agent's potential efficacy in the treatment of human erectile dysfunction.
  - The spinal cord
    - Guliano and associates have shown spinal cord involvement with dopamine as an erectogenic agent with intrathecal injection via catheter.[9]
    - These results suggest that there may be a dopamine spinal component in the control of penile erection.

Nitric Oxide

- Nitric oxide (NO) plays an important role in erectile function, both centrally and locally at the level of the penis.
- In the central nervous system, particularly in the paraventricular nucleus, NO serves as a positive mediator of erectile function.

- An increase in the production of NO in the hypothalamus is related to the positive effect of erections associated with administration of apomorphine.
- At the level of the corpora cavernosa, nitric oxide facilitates relaxation of the smooth muscle of the cavernosal arterioles. This action promotes the filling with blood of these arterioles, which raises the pressure within the corpora cavernosa. This leads to closure of the emissary veins, further promoting the process of erection.

Oxytocin

- Oxytocin may play an inhibitory role in erectile function.
  - Melis and colleagues have shown that penile erections induced by NO delivery in the paraventricular nucleus can be blocked by an oxytocin antagonist.[10]
  - On the other hand, Melis and colleagues have shown that oxytocin can induce penile erections in rats when injected bilaterally into the CA1 field of the hippocampus. However, the physiological importance of this strong cerebral role for oxytocin may be relative, as similar effects have not been demonstrated when oxytocin is administered peripherally.

Adrenocorticotropin (ACTH)

- Adrenocorticotropin (ACTH) has been shown to produce sexual excitation in several animal species.
- This peptide is derived from proopiomelanocortin and is expressed in the pituitary, hypothalamus, and brainstem.
- Serra and associates have shown that intracerebral injection of ACTH can induce penile erection and yawning behavior in rats.[11]
  - This group administered ACTH1-24 (3–5 micrograms/rat) and identified a behavioral syndrome characterized by recurrent episodes of penile erection and yawning in the rats.
  - On the other hand, in rats that underwent hypophysectomy, the ACTH1-24-induced yawning and penile erection was prevented.

- These results suggest that the pituitary has a "trophic" action, not only on peripheral target organs but also on structures in the brain that control specific behavioral responses.

Melanocyte-Stimulating Hormone (MSH)

■ Melanocyte-stimulating hormone (MSH), like ACTH, has been shown to produce sexual excitation in monkeys, rabbits, and rats.

■ This peptide is derived from proopiomelanocortin and is expressed in the pituitary, hypothalamus, and brainstem.

■ As with ACTH (as demonstrated by the work of Serra and associates), intracerebral injection of MSH not only induces penile erection in rats but also stimulates yawning behavior.

■ Wessels and colleagues studied an MSH analog compound known as Melanotan II, which underwent preliminary clinical trials as a potential agent for the treatment of erectile dysfunction.[12]

  - In this study, 10 subjects were enrolled in a double-blind, placebo-controlled crossover study.

  - Melanotan II (0.025 mg/kg) and vehicle were each administered twice by subcutaneous injection; real-time RigiScan monitoring and a visual analog were used to quantify the erections during a 6-hour period.

  - Melanotan II initiated subjectively reported erections in 12 of 19 injections versus only 1 of 21 doses of placebo. Nausea and stretching/yawning occurred more frequently with Melanotan II, and 4 of 19 injections were associated with severe nausea.

  - This agent has not been approved by the FDA for the treatment of erectile dysfunction because of the severe nausea in 20% of patients as well as the lack of demonstrated efficacy of this agent.

Androgen Control of Sexuality

■ Studies of patients who have undergone castration suggest that a decrease in male sexuality will occur.

- This is seen in patients who undergo radical orchiectomy for the treatment of hormone refractory prostate cancer.
- The resultant loss of testosterone after castration suggests the importance of androgens on sexual drive, motivation, and erectile function.
  - However, there are some caveats to consider.
    - There is no clearcut correlation between serum testosterone levels and erectile function. While castration results in impaired erectile function in most men, there are some men who are able to maintain erectile function despite castrate levels of testosterone.
    - On the other hand, not all men who have low levels of testosterone will have an improvement of their erectile function when they receive testosterone supplementation.
    - Androgens bind to a variety of sites within the brain, including the medial preoptic area, the amygdala, and the hypothalamus. It is also likely the androgens can interfere with other hormonal functions to impair sexuality. Androgens can impair the serotonin system, which may impair sexual function and behavior.

■ Conclusions

- Penile erection results from activation of autonomic nervous system with involvement of the sympathetic and parasympathetic systems.
- Multiple aminergic agents such as serotonin, norepinephrine, dopamine, nitric oxide, oxytocin, ACTH, and MSH play important roles in sexual dysfunction. As such, each of these compounds may play a role in male and female sexual dysfunction. Details regarding the pathophysiology of sexual dysfunction and treatment will be discussed in subsequent chapters.

■ Physiology of Ejaculation

- Orgasm and ejaculation complete the sexual response cycle.

- Ejaculation is a reflex involving multiple receptors and pathways.
- Ejaculation is controlled by a variety of hormonal forces, such as:
  - Serotonin
  - Dopamine
  - Cholinergic
  - Adrenergic
  - Oxytocin
  - GABA
- There are three basic mechanisms involved in normal antegrade ejaculation, as described in **Table 1.2**.
- Emission is the first mechanism of normal ejaculation.
  - Emission occurs due to sympathetic spinal cord reflex initiated by genital stimulation.
  - Contraction of the accessory sexual organs (seminal vesicles) occurs, leading to distension of the prostatic urethra.
  - This mechanism has considerable voluntary control initially, but with an increase in sensation, a point of inevitability of ejaculation is reached.

Table 1.2 Key Features of the Three Mechanisms of Normal Ejaculation

Emission
• Sympathetic spinal cord reflex
• Initiated by erotic stimuli
• Significant voluntary control
• Contraction of seminal vesicles and accessory sexual glands

Ejection
• Sympathetic spinal cord reflex
• Some voluntary control
• Pelvic floor muscle contractions
• External urethral sphincter relaxation

Orgasm
• Pressure builds up in posterior urethra
• Involuntary control
• Urethra contraction dispels ejaculate in antegrade manner

- Ejection is the second mechanism of normal ejaculation.
  - Ejection also involves significant sympathetic neural control.
  - Voluntary control in this phase is more limited.
  - The following physiological responses occur:
    - Closure of the bladder neck to prevent retrograde flow of ejaculate.
    - Contraction of the pelvic floor musculature (ischiocavernosus and bulbocavernosus muscles).
    - Relaxation of the urethral sphincter.
- Orgasm is the final mechanism of normal antegrade ejaculation.
  - Pudendal nerve stimulation occurs due to increased pressure in the posterior urethra. This pressure is ultimately released with contraction of the urethral bulb and accessory sexual organs.
- The ejaculate can be divided into several components, as shown in **Table 1.3**. The secretions that comprise the ejaculate come from:
  - The seminal vesicles (approximately 50–80% of the ejaculate volume)
  - Prostate gland (15–30% of the ejaculate volume)
  - Bulbourethral (Cowper) glands (less than 1% of the ejaculate volume)
  - Spermatozoa (less than 0.1% of the ejaculate volume)

◼ Hormonal Control of Ejaculation

- There are multiple neurochemical factors that may play a role in stimulating or inhibiting ejaculation. While dopamine and serotonin likely play dominant roles, the contributions of GABA and the cholinergic and adrenergic nervous systems have associated roles, as described as follows.

Table 1.3   Normal Contributions to Ejaculate Volume

Seminal vesicles	50–80%
Prostate gland secretions	15–30%
Bulbourethral (Cowper) gland secretions	3–5%
Spermatozoa	< 1%

Dopamine

- We have discussed previously the important role of dopamine in facilitating sexual behavior in rats. The works of Uitti and colleagues and Melis and colleagues demonstrate this rather well. It is also felt that the relative concentrations, or balance, between dopamine and serotonin further contribute to sexuality.
- On the receptor level, there are two families of dopamine receptors, known as D1 and D2.
  - The D2 family is important in drug therapy and there may be a modulatory effect by the D1 receptor on the D2 receptors. It is believed that dopamine via the D2 receptors promotes ejaculation. Serotonin, on the other hand, appears to inhibit ejaculation.
- It has been shown that altering this balance with selective serotonin reuptake inhibitors (SSRI) may prolong ejaculation.
  - This has lead to these agents being used in the treatment of premature ejaculation.
- Further studies by Hull and associates have suggested a possible sexual response regulatory role of dopamine.[13]
  - This is suggested by the observation that dopamine is released in the medial preoptic area of male rats in the presence of a hormonally active female rat. This causes ejaculation in the male rat.

Serotonin

- As mentioned previously, serotonin has an inhibitory effect on ejaculation.
- Serotonin is a vasoconstrictor, is identified in the blood and is predominantly located in the enterocromuffin cells of the gastrointestinal tract.
- Several 5-HT receptors have been identified and have been divided into classes.
  - The 5-HT1A receptor is thought to facilitate sexual behavior and can decrease ejaculatory latency time.
  - The 5-HT1B receptor is thought to inhibit ejaculatory behavior.
    - This has been shown by Ahlenius and collegues. In their study utilizing rats, the increased

ejaculatory latency produced by 5-HTP was blocked by treatment with isamoltane, a 5-HT1B receptor antagonist.

■ The brain serotonin system has an inhibitory role in sexuality and ejaculation in rats.

- This compound is released from the hypothalamus in male rats at the time of ejaculation.
- This inhibition of ejaculation also inhibits copulatory behavior as demonstrated by Lorrain and colleagues.[14]

Gamma-Aminobutyric Acid (GABA)

■ Gamma-aminobutyric acid (GABA) may play an inhibitory role in sexual functioning.

■ There are two types of GABA receptors:
- GABA-A
- GABA-B

■ Approximately 30–40% of neurons in the brain use GABA as their primary neurotransmitter.

■ Both receptor types appear to have an inhibitory response to sexual behavior.

■ Benzodiazepines, as a class, enhance GABA activity.

■ Qureshi and colleagues have shown that GABA inhibits sexual behavior in female rats.[15]

- They showed that postejaculatory suppression of sexual receptivity in female rats was partially reversed by intracerebroventricular injection of the GABA antagonist bicuculline and the behavior of receptive rats was inhibited by intracerebroventricular injection of the GABA agonist muscimol.
- Further, they showed that increasing the concentration of GABA in the cerebrospinal fluid by injection of the GABA transaminase inhibitor gamma-vinyl GABA caused an increase of the concentration of GABA in the cerebrospinal fluid and inhibited the display of sexual receptivity.

Cholinergic Nervous System

■ Cholinergic receptors are divided into two classes:
- Nicotinic
- Muscarinic

- The nicotinic receptor is located predominantly at the neuromuscular junction.
- When nicotinic receptor blockers are administered, an elevation of levels of serotonin in the brain is observed. Thus, administration of cholinergic blockers such as atropine will elevate serotonin levels and inhibit sexual behavior.
  - Bitran and colleagues have shown that microinjection of the cholinergic blocker scopolamine into the ventricles of the rat brain prolongs sexual behavior and increases the time to ejaculation in those rats.[16]

Adrenergic Nervous System

- Adrenergic control of erection and ejaculation occurs peripherally and centrally.
- In the central nervous system, there are alpha-receptors in the brain, while there are beta 1– and beta 2–receptors in the cortex and cerebellum.
- There is likely an important balance between adrenergic and cholinergic control of sexual function.
  - This balance likely explains the condition of priapism, which is a prolonged erection unrelated to sexual stimulation. This condition results from prolonged alpha-adrenergic blockade.
    - Seagraves and associates have shown than prazosin results in competitive antagonism of postsynaptic alpha 1–adrenergic receptors in tissues that sustain high levels of alpha-adrenergic sympathetic tone, leading to priapism.[17]

Nitric Oxide

- Nitric oxide (NO) is an important messenger in the brain.
- NO regulates emotional and sexual behavior.
  - Lorrain and associates have shown that nitric oxide facilitates copulatory behavior in rats by increasing dopamine release.[18]
    - In their study, local administration of the NO precursor L-arginine to rats also increased dopamine release in the medial preoptic area.

- Males received either NO synthesis inhibitor, nitro-L-arginine methyl ester (L-NAME, 400 μM), or its inactive isomer, D-NAME (400 μM), in the medial preoptic area via a microdialysis probe for 3 hours prior to the introduction of a female.
- Following D-NAME administration, dopamine increased during copulation, while L-NAME prevented this increase.
- Therefore, NO may promote dopamine release in the medial preoptic area of male rats, thereby facilitating copulation.

■ Conclusions

- Evidence concerning pharmacological effects on human sexuality suggests that dopaminergic receptor activation may be associated with penile erection.
- Erection also appears to involve inhibition of alpha-adrenergic influences and beta-adrenergic stimulation plus the release of a noncholinergic vasodilator substance, possibly vasoactive intestinal peptide.
- Ejaculation appears to be mediated primarily by alpha-adrenergic fibers. Serotonergic neurotransmission may inhibit the ejaculatory reflex.
- An understanding of the neurobiological substrate of human sexuality may assist clinicians in choosing psychotropic agents with minimal adverse effects on sexual behavior and may also contribute to the development of pharmacological interventions for sexual difficulties.

■ References

1. Johnson RD, Hubscher CH. Brainstem microstimulation differentially inhibits pudendal motoneuron reflex inputs. *Brain Res.* 1984;302:315–321.
2. Ahlenius S, Larrson K. Evidence for involvement of 5-HT1B receptors in the inhibition of male rat ejaculatory behavior by 5-HTP. *Psychopharmacology* (Berl). 1998;137:374–382.
3. Yaici D, Rampin O, Calas A, et al. Alpha(2a) and alpha(2c) adrenoreceptors on spinal neurons controlling penile erection. *Neuroscience.* 2002;114:945–960.

4. Kaplan SA, Reis RB, Kohn IJ, et al. Combination therapy using oral alpha blockers and intracavernosal injection in men with erectile dysfunction. *Urology* 1998;52:739–743.

5. Morales A. Yohimbine in erectile dysfunction: the facts. *Int J Impot Res.* 2000;12(S1):S70–S74.

6. Ernst E, Pittler MH. Yohimbine for erectile dysfunction: a systematic review and meta-analysis of randomized clinical trials. *J Urol.* 1998;159:433–436.

7. Uitti RJ, Tanner CM, Rajput AH, et al. Hypersexuality with antiparkinsonian therapy. *Clin Neuropharmacol.* 1989;12:375–383.

8. Melis MR, Argiolas A, Gessa GL. Apomorphine-induced penile erection and yawning: site of action in brain. *Brain Res.* 1987;415:98–104.

9. Guliano F, Allard J, Bernabe J, et al. Spinal proerectile effect of apomorphine in the anesthetized rat. *Int J Impot Res.* 2001; 13:110–115.

10. Melis MR, Argiolas A. Nitric oxide donors induce penile erection and yawning: site of action in the brain. *Brain Res.* 1986;398:259–265.

11. Serra G, Fratta W, Collu M, et al. Hypophysectomy prevents ACTH-induced yawning and penile erection in rats. *Pharmacol Biochem Behav.* 1987;26:277–279.

12. Wessels H, Gralnek D, Dorr R, et al. Effect of an alpha melanocyte stimulating hormone analog on penile erection and sexual desire in men with organic erectile dysfunction. *Urol.* 2000;56:641–646.

13. Hull EM, Du J, Lorrain DS, et al. Extracellular dopamine in the medial preoptic area: implications for sexual motivation and hormonal control of copulation. *Life Sci.* 1992;51:1705–1713.

14. Lorrain DS, Matuszewich L, Friedman RD, et al. Extracellular serotonin in the lateral hypothalamic area is increased during the postejaculatory period and impairs copulation in male rats. *J Neurosci.* 1997;17(23):9361–9366.

15. Qureshi GA, Bednar I, Forsberg G, et al. GABA inhibits sexual behavior in female rats. *Neuroscience.* 1988;27:169–174.

16. Bitran D, Hull EM. Pharmacologic analysis of male rat sexual behavior. *Neurosci Biobehav Rev.* 1987;11:365–389.

17. Seagraves RT. Effects of psychotropic drugs on human erection and ejaculation. *Arch Gen Psychiatry.* 1989;46:275–284.

18. Lorrain DS, Hull EM. Nitric oxide increases dopamine and serotonin release in the medial preoptic area. *Neuroreport.* 1996;8:31–34.

CHAPTER 2

Pathophysiology of Erectile Dysfunction

Aimee Rogers, MD ■ *Stanley Zaslau, MD, MBA, FACS*

■ Introduction

- Erectile dysfunction (ED) is defined according to the National Institute of Health consensus development panel as the persistent inability to attain and/or maintain an erection sufficient to permit satisfactory sexual intercourse.[1]
- The ED must cause some degree of personal distress either to the patient himself or to the couple before treatment should be considered.
- ED is believed to be a subjective condition.
- This chapter will review the pathophysiology of ED.
  - First, a discussion of the epidemiology and incidence will be presented.
  - Next, we will classify erectile dysfunction according to a functional classification.
  - Finally, we will review the association of ED to systemic diseases such as diabetes mellitus, hyperlipidemia, atherosclerosis, hypertension, renal failure, and psychogenic causes.

■ Epidemiology

- One of the most important epidemiological studies on ED is the Massachusetts Male Aging Study.
  - In this study, Feldman and colleagues surveyed 1709 men between the ages of 40 and 70 utilizing a self-administered sexual function questionnaire.[2]
  - This random-sample, community-based survey indicated that the overall mean probability of having some degree of sexual dysfunction was 52%. As a man ages

from 40 to 70 years of age, his likelihood of having complete ED triples from approximately 5% to 15%. Also during this time period, the likelihood of having moderate ED doubles from 17% to 34%. However, the likelihood of having mild ED was 17% and remained that way throughout the time period.

- Age was found to be the most important independent predictor of ED. In addition, diabetes mellitus, hypertension, and heart disease were also significant predictors of ED. Interestingly, smoking and alcohol consumption were only weakly correlated with ED.

■ The Olmstead County Study by Panser and colleagues showed similar results between aging and ED.[3]

- In this study of 2115 men aged 40 to 70 years, the prevalence of ED increased from 12.6% between ages 40 and 49 to 25% between ages 70 and 79. Only 18% of men over the age of 70 were usually able to obtain an erection. Approximately 25% of men over the age of 70 were unable to have an erection at all.

■ Johannes and colleagues evaluated 847 men from the Massachusetts Male Aging Study who were without erectile dysfunction at baseline and had completed the study.[4]

- Erectile dysfunction was assessed by a self-administered sexual function questionnaire and a single global self-rating question.

- Researchers found that the crude incidence rate for erectile dysfunction was 25.9 cases per 1000 man-years. The annual incidence rate increased with each decade of age and was 12.4 cases per 1000 man-years for men ages 40 to 49, 29.8 for men ages 50 to 59, and 46.4 for men ages 60 to 69.

- The age-adjusted risk of erectile dysfunction was higher for men with lower education, diabetes, heart disease, and hypertension.

■ Classification

■ Many classifications have been proposed for ED. Some systems are based on cause of ED (e.g., diabetes, trauma), while others are based on the neurovascular mechanism of the erectile process (e.g., neurogenic, vasculogenic, arterial, venous).

■ Lizza and colleagues, through the International Society for the Study of Impotence Research, developed a simple classification system for ED. We will discuss this classification system in detail as follows.[5]

  • An outline of the classification system is presented in **Table 2.1**.

Psychogenic

■ In years past, psychogenic ED was felt to be the most common type.

  • In fact, in 1970, Masters and Johnson believed that this represented 90% of cases of ED.[6]

■ However, at present, researchers believe that most men with ED have a mixed condition, with a predominantly functional component and some secondary associated psychogenic component.

■ In addition, a number of other factors should be considered that contribute to this form of ED, including:

  • Deterioration of the relationship between partners
  • Job loss
  • Loss of partner
  • Health problems of patient and partner

■ These problems can lead to anger, hostility, alienation of one's partner, and/or the partner not being interested in intimacy. Thus, it becomes difficult for a man to obtain a functional erection under these circumstances.

Table 2.1   Classification of Male Erectile Dysfunction

Organic causes
Vasculogenic
Arteriogenic
Cavernosal
Mixed
Neurogenic
Anatomic
Endocrinologic
Psychogenic causes

- Further, life-altering situations, such as death of a spouse, can lead to personal stresses such as guilt, anger, and confusion, which can impair erectile function.

Neurogenic

- As mentioned previously, erectile function normally requires an intact vascular system and neurological system. Thus, impairment of the neurological system can result in changes in erectile function.

- As previously discussed, the neural relationships between the brain, spinal cord, and cavernosal nerves are important. As such, diseases in these areas can impair erectile function.

- At the central nervous system level, numerous diseases such as cerebrovascular accident, Parkinson's disease, and Alzheimer's disease can result in ED.

- As mentioned previously, the dopaminergic nervous system also plays an important role in erectile function. An imbalance in this system caused by dopamine antagonists can impair erectile function, as is often the case in patients with Parkinson's disease.

- Spinal cord injury can also result in ED. The type of ED is related to the location of the spinal cord injury.
  - Reflexogenic erections are preserved in patients who have lesions of the upper spinal cord.
  - However, patients with lumbar or sacral injuries often cannot obtain erections.
  - Other spinal cord disease states associated with erectile dysfunction include tumors of the spinal cord, spina bifida, syringomyelia, and multiple sclerosis.

- One of the most common causes of neurogenic erectile dysfunction occurs after radical prostatectomy due to damage to the cavernosal nerves.
  - Finkle and colleagues conducted a retrospective study of 62 patients who underwent radical prostatectomy with normal preoperative erectile function.[7]
    - Postoperatively, 43% reported normal erections and resumption of sexual intercourse.

- Preservation of potency after radical prostatectomy is related to several factors, including:
  - Age of the patient (younger patients tend to fare better than older patients)
  - Preoperative continence status (continent patients tend to fare better than incontinent patients)
  - Preservation of the neurovascular bundle (patients with one or both neurovascular bundles spared fare better than patients who have both neurovascular bundles transected).
- Weinstein and colleagues reported that following abdominoperineal resection, where the entire rectum was extirpated, the effect on sexual functioning differed for men and women.[8] Sexual function in men was completely destroyed, while women were capable of continuing sexual enjoyment as before the operation.
  - This suggests the importance of the parasympathetic fibers to male erectile function.
- Erectile dysfunction can also occur after endoscopic surgical procedures to the urethra.
  - McDermott and colleagues have shown impotence rates of up to 50% after cold knife urethrotomy procedures.[9]
- Pelvic fracture can result in ED due to pelvic and cavernosal nerve injury.
  - This can result from posterior urethral disruption because in this setting, injury to the puboprostatic ligament can dislodge the prostate from the posterior urethra.
  - This same force can result from cavernosal nerve injury. Patients can have ED after urethroplasty as a result of both the initial injury and the surgical attempt to reconstruct the urethra.

■ Endocrinologic

- Endocrinologic causes of ED can occur due to hypogonadism, hyperprolactinemia or thyroid disease. Hypogonadism is common in patients with ED.

- Hypogonadism can be associated with low serum testosterone levels. This condition is associated with:
  1. decreased sexual interest
  2. decreased frequency of sexual acts
  3. decreased frequency of nocturnal erections
- Granata and associates evaluated the relationship between nocturnal erections and testosterone levels in 201 men. They found that the threshold testosterone level for normal nocturnal erections is approximately 200 ng/dL.[10]
- In addition, dysfunction of the hypothalamic-pituitary axis can result in hypogonadism and ED. Disorders such as hypogonadotrophic hypogonadism can be due to tumors or injury.
- In addition, hypergonotrophic hypogonadism can be due to tumor, testicular injury or viral causes such as mumps orchitis.
- Hyperprolactinemia can also result in ED. This can be due to pituitary tumors or medications. Patients may present with ED, galactorrhea, gynecomastia and unexplained male infertility.
- Leonard and colleagues evaluated 1236 consecutive impotent patients and found elevated serum prolactin levels in approximately 6%. These patients also had low levels of serum testosterone.[11]
- Patients with hyperthyroidism can also have ED. Symptoms of hyperthyroidism include decreased libido, which is often associated with increased serum estrogen levels.
- On the other hand, patients with hypothyroidism often have low serum testosterone and elevated prolactin levels. Thus, both thyroid hyper- or hypo-functioning states can be associated with ED.

■ Arteriogenic

- Arteriogenic ED can be due to a variety of reasons including trauma to the hypogastric, cavernosal, or helicine arteries or due to atherosclerotic disease. These diseases result in decreased penile perfusion.

- Risk factors for arterial insufficiency include:
  1. hypertension
  2. hyperlipidemia
  3. cigarette smoking
  4. diabetes mellitus
  5. blunt perineal or pelvic trauma
  6. pelvic irradiation
- Arteriography studies, although not commonly performed, indicate some important findings: Patients with atherosclerosis typically have diffuse bilateral disease of the internal pudendal, common penile, and/or cavernosal arteries.
- Levine and colleagues reviewed the results of 24 male patients with blunt pelvic or perineal trauma who developed immediate impotence. This group found that blunt pelvic trauma was associated with a higher incidence of the distal internal or common penile artery injuries.[12]
- Ruzbarsky and colleagues did postmortem studies of the arterial bed in 15 male diabetics. They found fibrous proliferation of the intima, medial fibrosis, calcification, and narrowing of the lumen to obliteration from thrombi. The extent of the pathology was apparently related to both age and diabetes mellitus. This certainly explains the high incidence of ED in this population.[13]
- Finally, ED and cardiovascular disease share the same risk factors such as hypertension, diabetes mellitus, hypercholesterolemia and smoking. As such, ED can be a presenting or accompanying symptom in these conditions.

■ Vasculogenic

- Venogenic erectile dysfunction results from a variety of reasons including failure of the veno-occlusive mechanism. The following mechanisms further explain this dysfunction:
  1. Dilation of the venous channels in the corpora cavernosa
  2. Inadequate compression of the emmissary veins due to underlying disease. Example:
     Peyronie's Disease due to the fibrous scarring of the tunica albiguinea can prevent adequate emissary vein closure.

3. Smooth muscle dysfunction within the cavernosal vasculature can lead to venous leakage. This can be associated with impaired nitric oxide release and impair corporal smooth muscle relaxation.

4. Patients who have a history of priapism and had undergone an arterio-venous shunt will have presistent venous leakage due to this prior shunt.

■ There are four components of venogenic ED to consider further:

- Fibroelastic component
- Smooth muscle
- Gap junctions
- Endothelium

  - *The fibroelastic component.* With development of diseases such as diabetes, hypercholesterolemia and aging, there is loss of compliance of the penile sinusoids. Collagen deposition occurs.

  - *The smooth muscle component.* Relaxation of corporal smooth muscle leads to erection. Thus, conditions which damage the corporal smooth muscle will be associated with erectile dysfunction. Thus, patients with diabetes have damage to the vascular smooth muscle in the cavernosal tissues. This smooth muscle disease has micro level dysfunction as well. Alteration of normal ion channels can occur. Specifically, deficits in ion transport of potassium and calcium are likely. Because of these deficits, altered smooth muscle calcium homeostasis occurs leading to impaired relaxation of the cavernosal smooth muscle tissue in patients with ED.

  - *The gap junction component.* The gap junctions are responsible for communication between cells and plays an important role in the regulation of the normal erectile process. It is possible that in patients with severe vascular disease that normal cavernosal cells lose their ability to contact each other because of the fibrosis that develops between cells. This can lead to a lack of coordinated relaxation of cavernosal smooth muscle cells.

- *The endothelial component.* The normal endothelium functions to promote erections and flaccidity through the release of prostglandins, endothelins and nitric oxide. This is due to mediation through the cholinergic and adrenergic nervous systems. Various disease states have been known to impair nitric oxide release and endothelium-mediated relaxation of the cavernosal smooth muscle tissue. Impairment of this mechanism occurs in diabetes and hypercholesterolemia.

■ Conclusions

- Practitioners should remember that many classifications have been proposed for ED. Some systems are based on cause of ED (e.g., diabetes, trauma), while others are based on the neurovascular mechanism of the erectile process (e.g., neurogenic, vasculogenic, arterial, venous).
- There are many conditions that can contribute to ED. These can be organic and/or psychologic.
- Our understanding of the development and treatment of ED continues to evolve.

■ References

1. NIH consensus development panel on impotence. *JAMA.* 1993;27:83–90.

2. Feldman HA, Goldstein I, Hatzichristou DG, et al. Impotence and its medical and psychological correlates: results of the Massachusetts Male Aging Study. *J Urol.* 1994;151:54–61.

3. Panser LA, Rhodes T, Girman CJ, et al. Sexual function of men age 40 to 79 years: the Olmstead County Study of Urinary Symptoms and Health Status Among Men. *J Am Geriatr Soc.* 1995;43(10):1107–1110.

4. Johannes CB, Araujo AB, Feldman HA, et al. Incidence of erectile dysfunction in men ages 40–69: longitudinal results from the Massachusetts Male Aging Study. *J Urol.* 2000;163:460.

5. Lizza EF, Rosen RC. Definition and classification of erectile dysfunction: report of the Nomenclature Committee of

the International Society of Impotence Research. *Int J Impot Res.* 1999;11:141.

6. Masters W, Johnson V. *Human Sexual Response.* Boston, MA: Little-Brown; 1970.

7. Finkle AL, Taylor SP. Sexual potency after radical prostatectomy. *J Urol.* 1981;125:350.

8. Weinstein M, Roberts M. Sexual potency following surgery for rectal carcinoma. A follow-up of 44 patients. *Ann Surg.* 1977;185:295.

9. McDermott DW, Bates RJ, Heney NM, et al. Erectile impotence as a complication of direct vision cold knife urethrotomy. *Urology.* 1981;18:467.

10. Granata AR, Rochira V, Lerchl A, et al. Relationship between sleep-related erections and testosterone levels in men. *J Androl.* 1997;18:522–527.

11. Leonard MJ, Nickel CJ, Morales A. Hyperprolactinemia and impotence: why, when and how to investigate. *J Urol.* 1989;142:992–994.

12. Levine FJ, Greenfield AJ, Goldstein I. Arteriographically determined occlusive disease within the hypogastric-cavernous bed in impotent patients following blunt and perineal and pelvic trauma. *J Urol.* 1990;144:1147–1153.

13. Ruzbarsky V, Michal V. Morphological changes in the arterial bed of the penis with aging. Relationship to the pathogenesis of impotence. *Invest Urol.* 1977; Nov 15(3):194–199.

CHAPTER 3

Physical Diagnosis and Testing

Aimee E. Rogers, MD ■ *Stanley Zaslau, MD, MBA, FACS*

■ Introduction

- There are many components to a successful sexual act, and dysfunction can occur at any point in the process.
- The sexually competent male must:
  - Have desire for his sexual partner (libido)
  - Direct blood from the iliac artery into the corpora cavernosa to achieve penile tumescence and rigidity (erection) adequate for penetration
  - Discharge sperm and prostatic/seminal vesicle fluid through the urethra (ejaculation)
  - Experience a sense of pleasure (orgasm)[1]
- At any point in time, this process can break down, which results in erectile dysfunction. This can be due to:
  - Psychological causes
  - Medications
  - Hormonal abnormalities
  - Neurological issues
  - Vasculopathy
- Those issues and the other various etiologies of male sexual dysfunction will be discussed separately. This chapter will focus on physical diagnosis and evaluation of erectile dysfunction with the use of an ever-expanding array of tools, ranging from questionnaires and Doppler ultrasounds to penile arterial blood flow mapping.

■ Initial Evaluation

- The evaluation begins with a sexual history and physical examination. The history and physical examination have been reported to have a 95% sensitivity, but only a 50% specificity in determining the cause of impotence; as a result, additional diagnostic tests are needed to maximize specificity.[2]

- The sexual history includes important information such as:
  - Rapidity of onset of dysfunction
  - Duration of dysfunction
  - Severity of the problem
  - An assessment of risk factors for impotence
- Sexually competent men who suddenly develop symptoms 'overnight' are usually those who have a psychogenic component to their sexual dysfunction.
  - This is contrasted with men who notice their sexual function fail sporadically, then worsen over time. These men are likely suffering from organic disease, whether it be neurogenic or vascular.
- Another important component of the sexual history is erectile reserve. In men presenting with erectile dysfunction, the presence or absence of spontaneous erections is an important clue to diagnosis.
  - Most men experience spontaneous erections during REM sleep, and often wake up with an erection, attesting to the integrity of neurogenic reflexes and corpora cavernosa blood flow.[3] Reports of either morning or nocturnal erections can usually be elicited by either the patient or his partner.
  - Men who report the lack of either type of spontaneous erection usually suffer from either neurological or vascular disease.
- It's also important to remember the importance of the patient's medical history.
- According to Lue and Broderick, the goals of medical history taking are:
  - To evaluate the potential role of underlying medical conditions (e.g., atherosclerosis, diabetes) and comorbidities (e.g., depression)
  - To differentiate between potential organic and psychogenic causes

- To assess the potential role of medication-induced ED
  - With respect to the final goal of history taking, it is important to remember that some medications, such as some beta-blockers, may contribute to the patient's sexual dysfunction, and some, such as nitrates, may be contraindicated for use in treatment of erectile dysfunction.[4]
- The physical examination begins with assessment of the heart, lungs, and abdomen. In addition to the basic physical examination, the evaluation of the sexually dysfunctional male should include the following:
  - Evaluation of body habitus and an assessment of secondary sexual characteristics
  - A careful assessment of femoral and peripheral pulses as a clue to the presence of vasculogenic disease
  - A breast examination to evaluate for possible gynecomastia, indicative of certain genetic syndromes
  - Examination of the testicles, noting any atrophy, asymmetry, or masses
  - A thorough examination of the penis, looking for evidence of chordee, micropenis, or Peyronie's plaque
  - Testing for genital and perineal sensation, and eliciting the bulbocavernosus reflex (BCR)
  - Testing for visual field defects, indicative of a pituitary tumor with resultant hypogonadism
- A patient's past surgical history may similarly yield insights. Radical pelvic surgery (e.g., prostatectomy, abdominoperineal resection) and pelvic trauma are well known to be associated with erectile dysfunction.[5,6]

◼ Laboratory Testing

- Laboratory tests for men with sexual dysfunction usually start with a fasting glucose and lipid profile to assess for any potential medical comorbidities, such as diabetes or hyperlipidemia.
- This is usually followed closely by hormonal profiles, including serum testosterone, prolactin, and thyroid function tests.

- A majority of the time, male sexual dysfunction that stems from a hormonal abnormality is a result of testosterone deficiency, or hypogonadism.
  - Hypogonadism in a male refers to a decrease in one or both of the two major functions of the testes: sperm production or testosterone production.[7]
  - These abnormalities can result from dysfunction of the testes, as in primary hypogonadism, or from pituitary or hypothalamic dysfunction, as seen in secondary hypogonadism.
  - If the testosterone level is below or at the low limit of normal, the practitioner should then obtain serum concentrations of luteinizing hormone (LH) and follicle-stimulating hormone (FSH). These values allow differentiation between primary (above-normal FSH/LH) hypogonadism and secondary (normal or reduced FSH/LH) hypogonadism.
- A prolactin level is drawn to rule out any possible dysfunction of the hypothalamic-pituitary axis.
  - False elevations of prolactin levels can be seen after large meals, stress, or certain types of drugs.
  - Any man with a confirmed diagnosis of hyperprolactinemia (non-drug-induced) should undergo investigation of the hypothalamic-pituitary axis, preferably an MRI, to rule out the presence of a tumor responsible for the hyperprolactinemia.[8]
- Thyroid function tests are usually performed in order to rule out hyper- or hypothyroidism as a cause of the patient's sexual dysfunction.
  - In men with hyperthyroidism, an increase in serum SHBG concentrations results in high serum total testosterone concentrations, but serum-free (unbound) testosterone concentrations are normal or low.[9]
  - Extragonadal conversion of testosterone to estradiol is increased, which results in elevated serum estradiol concentrations.
  - According to Carani et al., these changes can cause:
    - Gynecomastia
    - Reduced libido
    - Erectile dysfunction[10]

- The same authors found that hypothyroidism also has a negative effect on sexual function. They found that 64% of hypothyroid men evaluated in their multicenter prospective study experienced decreased libido, erectile dysfunction, and delayed ejaculation.

■ Noninvasive Methods of Evaluation

- After the history and physical exam are completed, the practitioner's attention should turn to the noninvasive methods of evaluation of erectile dysfunction.
- This is most commonly in the form of questionnaires and sexual function symptom scores.
  - Many ED questionnaires and sexual function profiles have been developed over the years.
  - They were initially used to differentiate psychogenic ED from nonpsychogenic ED.
  - More recently, a variety of self-report measures for assessing the levels of male sexual function or dysfunction have been created; self-administered questionnaires (SAQs) have seen their greatest use in clinical trials.
  - SAQs attempt to quantify sexual interest, performance, and satisfaction.
    - The most commonly referenced SAQs include:
      - The International Index of Erectile Function (IIEF) by Rosen and associates (1997)
      - The Brief Male Sexual Function Inventory (BMSFI) by O'Leary and colleagues (1995)
      - The Erectile Dysfunction Inventory for Treatment Satisfaction (EDITS) by Althof and associates (1999)[11]
    - The IIEF is the most widely used SAQ, and it is statistically validated in many languages. Its items address and quantify five domains:
      - Erectile function
      - Orgasmic function
      - Sexual desire
      - Intercourse satisfaction
      - Overall satisfaction[12]

- It is important to remember that all sexual inventories rely on self-assessment.
  - In 1999, Blander and colleagues demonstrated that SAQs do not differentiate among the various causes of ED (vascular, neurogenic, or psychogenic), and evidence-based assessments such as diagnostic tests are still necessary in patients with complex erectile dysfunction.[13]
- Nocturnal penile tumescence (NPT) testing was first described in 1940 by Halverson, who documented nocturnal erections in infants.
  - In 1966, Karacan and colleagues were the first to demonstrate that 80% of NPT occurs during rapid eye movement (REM) sleep.
  - Total tumescence time during sleep peaks during puberty, when as much as 20% of total sleep time may be spent with an erection.
  - In the second decade of life, the average duration of nocturnal erection is 38 minutes. In adults, the average duration of the erectile state is 27 minutes.[14]
  - NPT was initially used by psychologists to study sleep and dreams. Fairly recently, it has been applied to differentiate psychogenic from organic erectile dysfunction.
  - Historically, NPT has been measured by a variety of methods.
    - The earliest methods include:
      - The stamp test (Barry et al., 1980)
      - Snap gauges (Diedrich et al., 1992)
      - Sleep laboratory nocturnal penile tumescence and rigidity (NPTR)
    - The RigiScan (Endocare, Inc., Irvine, California) was introduced in 1985, and it was the first device to provide automated, portable NPT recording.
    - Most recently, NPT electrobioimpedance (NEVA American Medical Systems, Inc., Minnetonka, Minnesota) testing has been introduced as the most advanced form of nocturnal penile tumescence testing.

- In its most classic form, NPT consists of nocturnal monitoring devices that measure:
  - The number of erectile episodes
  - Tumescence (circumference change by strain gauges)
  - Maximal penile rigidity
  - Duration of nocturnal erections[15]
- Traditionally, NPT was recorded in conjunction with various other monitoring devices, including electro-encephalography, electro-oculography, electromyography (EMG), and oxygen saturation measurements to document REM sleep and the presence or absence of sleep apnea.
  - In these evaluations, the patient is awakened during maximal tumescence, and the erection is photographed and axial rigidity measured with a device applied to the tip of the penis.
- In the past, formal NPT evaluations were costly because they needed to be conducted in specially equipped sleep centers with trained observers.[16] Recently, NPT testing has been simplified.
- Devices such as the RigiScan provide accurate, reproducible information quantifying the number, duration, tumescence, and radial rigidity of erectile episodes a man experiences as he sleeps in the comfort of his own bed.[17]
  - The RigiScan consists of a recording unit that collects data for three separate nights for a maximum of 10 hours each night.
  - The device consists of two loops.
    - One is placed at the base of the penis.
    - The other is placed at the coronal sulcus.
  - Via constriction of the loops, the device records penile tumescence (circumference) and radial rigidity at the penile base and tip.
  - A baseline penile circumference is established while the patient is awake prior to the test.
  - Penile rigidity is recorded every three minutes by constriction of the loops. If the loop at the base

detects a circumference increase of greater than
10mm, sampling is increased to every 30 seconds.[18]

- The data generated can be downloaded to provide a
  graphic index quantifying erectile activity as either
  normal or impaired.
- Radial rigidity above 70% represents a nonbuckling
  erection, and a rigidity of less than 40% represents
  a flaccid penis.

- According to Levine's study of NPT, the number of erections considered normal is three to six per 8-hour session,
  lasting an average of 10 to 15 minutes each.[19]
- In 1992, Cilurzo and colleagues recommended the following as normal NPT recording criteria[20]:
  a. Four to five erectile episodes per night
  b. Mean duration of erection longer than 30 minutes
  c. An increase in circumference of more than 3 cm at
     the base and more than 2 cm at the tip
  d. Maximal rigidity above 70% at both base and tip

  As can be seen from the data presented by Levine[19] and
  Cilurzo[20] there is some variability as to normal NPT recording criteria.

  Men who are experiencing sexual dysfunction with a
  normal NPT are considered to have psychogenic erectile dysfunction, whereas those with impaired NPT are
  considered to have "organic" erectile dysfunction, usually
  due to vascular or neurological disease.
  a. In comparison, testosterone-deficient hypogonadal
     men are still capable of exhibiting some erectile ac-
     tivity during nocturnal penile tumescence studies.[21]

■ Vascular Evaluation

- Vascular evaluation is performed in men with erectile
  dysfunction in order to diagnose those with arterial and
  venous occlusive dysfunction.
- Over the years, multiple tests have been developed to
  identify and quantify arterial and veno-occlusive disease.
  - This includes:
    - Combined intracavernous injection and stimula-
      tion (CIS)

- Duplex ultrasound
- Dynamic infusion cavernosometry and cavernosography (DICC)
- Selective penile angiography

- Traditionally, the first-line evaluation of penile blood flow has been combined intracavernous injection and stimulation (CIS).
  - CIS consists of:
    - An intracavernous injection of a vasodilator or a combination of two or three vasodilators
    - Genital or audiovisual sexual stimulation
    - Assessment of the erection by an observer[22]
  - Several intracavernosal injection agents have been used, including:
    - Alprostadil alone (Caverject or Edex)
    - A combination of papaverine and phentolamine (Bimix)
    - A mixture of all three agents (Trimix)
  - The technique involves injecting the chosen medication into the corpus cavernosum. The erectile response is periodically evaluated for both rigidity and duration.
  - The CIS test is the most commonly performed diagnostic procedure for erectile dysfunction. It allows the clinician to bypass neurological and hormonal influences, and to evaluate the vascular status of the penis directly via observation.[23]
- The second-line evaluation of penile blood flow is usually duplex ultrasonography (grayscale or color-coded).

Duplex ultrasound consists of high-resolution, real-time ultrasonography and color-pulsed Doppler, which enables the ultrasonographer to visualize the dorsal and cavernous arteries selectively and to perform dynamic blood flow analysis. It is also the best tool available for the diagnosis of high-flow priapism and localization of a ruptured artery.[24]

■ Conclusions

- The initial evaluation of the patient with sexual dysfunction must include a thorough sexual history and physical examination.

- The physical examination has a very high sensitivity but a low specificity thus sometimes requiring additional diagnostic testing to confirm the diagnosis.
- It is important to rule out other silent, but coexisting conditions such as diabetes, and hyperlipidemia.
- Important noninvasive methods of evaluation of ED include questionnaires and sexual function symptom scores.

■ References

1. Spark RF. Evaluation of male sexual dysfunction. *UpToDate*. 2008.

2. Davis-Joseph B, Tiefer L, Melman A. Accuracy of the initial history and physical examination to establish the etiology of erectile dysfunction. *Urology*. 1995;45:498.

3. Spark RF. Evaluation of male sexual dysfunction. *UpToDate*. 2008.

4. Broderick GA, Lue TF. Evaluation and nonsurgical management of erectile dysfunction and premature ejaculation. In: Wein AJ, Kavoussi LR, Novick AC, Partin AW, Peters CA, eds. *Campbell-Walsh Urology*. Ninth ed. Philadelphia, PA: Saunders Elsevier Company; 2007:750–787.

5. Armenakas NA, McAninch JW, Lue TF, et al. Posttraumatic impotence: magnetic resonance imaging and duplex ultrasound in diagnosis and management. *J Urol*. 1993;149:1272–1275.

6. Walsh PC, Partin AW, Epstein JI. Cancer control and quality of life following anatomical radical retropubic prostatectomy: results at 10 years. *J Urol*. 1994;152:1831–1836.

7. Snyder, PJ. Clinical features and diagnosis of male hypogonadism. *UpToDate*. 2009.

8. Broderick GA, Lue TF. Evaluation and nonsurgical management of erectile dysfunction and premature ejaculation. In: Wein AJ, Kavoussi LR, Novick AC, Partin AW, Peters CA, eds. *Campbell-Walsh Urology*. Ninth ed. Philadelphia, PA: Saunders Elsevier Company; 2007:750–787.

9. Abalovich M, Levalle O, Hermes R, et al. Hypothalamic-pituitary-testicular axis and seminal parameters in hyperthyroid males. *Thyroid*. 1999;9:857.

10. Carani C, Isidori AM, Granata A, et al. Multicenter study on the prevalence of sexual symptoms in male

hypo- and hyperthyroid patients. *J Clin Endocrinol Metab.* 2005;90:6472.

11. Broderick GA, Lue TF. Evaluation and nonsurgical management of erectile dysfunction and premature ejaculation. In: Wein AJ, Kavoussi LR, Novick AC, Partin AW, Peters CA, eds. *Campbell-Walsh Urology.* Ninth ed. Philadelphia, PA: Saunders Elsevier Company; 2007:750–787.

12. Rosen RC, Riley A, Wagner G, et al. The international index of erectile function (IIEF): a multidimensional scale for assessment of erectile dysfunction. *Urology.* 1997; 49:822–830.

13. Blander DS, Sánchez-Ortiz RF, Broderick GA. Sex inventories: can questionnaires replace erectile dysfunction testing? *Urology.* 1999;54(4):719–723.

14. Karacan I, Williams RL, Finley WW, Hursch CJ. The effects of naps on nocturnal sleep: influence on the need for stage-1 REM and stage 4 sleep. *Biol Psychiatry.* 1970;2(4): 391–399.

15. Kessler WO. Nocturnal penile tumescence. *Urol Clin North Am.* 1988;15(1):81–86.

16. Broderick GA, Lue TF. Evaluation and nonsurgical management of erectile dysfunction and premature ejaculation. In: Wein AJ, Kavoussi LR, Novick AC, Partin AW, Peters CA, eds. *Campbell-Walsh Urology.* Ninth ed. Philadelphia, PA: Saunders Elsevier Company; 2007:750–787.

17. Bain CL, Guay AT. Reproducibility in measuring nocturnal penile tumescence and rigidity. *J Urol.* 1992;148:811.

18. Broderick GA, Lue TF. Evaluation and nonsurgical management of erectile dysfunction and premature ejaculation. In: Wein AJ, Kavoussi LR, Novick AC, Partin AW, Peters CA, eds. *Campbell-Walsh Urology.* Ninth ed. Philadelphia, PA: Saunders Elsevier Company; 2007:750–787.

19. Levine LA, Lenting EL. Use of nocturnal penile tumescence and rigidity in the evaluation of male erectile dysfunction. *Urol Clin North Am.* 1995;22(4):775–788.

20. Cilurzo P, Canale D, Turchi P, Giorgi PM, Menchini Fabris GF. The Rigiscan system in the diagnosis of male sexual impotence. *Arch Ital Urol Nefrol Androl.* 1992;64(S2): 81–85.

21. Kwan M, Greenleaf WJ, Mann J, et al. The nature of androgen action on male sexuality: a combined laboratory-self-report study on hypogonadal men. *J Clin Endocrinol Metab.* 1983;57:557.

22. Donatucci CF, Lue TF. The combined intracavernous injection and stimulation test: diagnostic accuracy. *J Urol.* 1992;148(1):61–62.
23. Broderick GA, Lue TF. Evaluation and nonsurgical management of erectile dysfunction and premature ejaculation. In: Wein AJ, Kavoussi LR, Novick AC, Partin AW, Peters CA, eds. *Campbell-Walsh Urology.* Ninth ed. Philadelphia, PA: Saunders Elsevier Company; 2007:750–787.
24. Broderick GA, Lue TF. Evaluation and nonsurgical management of erectile dysfunction and premature ejaculation. In: Wein AJ, Kavoussi LR, Novick AC, Partin AW, Peters CA, eds. *Campbell-Walsh Urology.* Ninth ed. Philadelphia, PA: Saunders Elsevier Company; 2007:750–787.

CHAPTER 4

Medical Therapies for Erectile Dysfunction

Adam Luchey, MD ■ *Stanley Zaslau, MD, MBA, FACS*

■ Introduction

- When considering treatment for sexual dysfunction, management is grouped into:
  - Erectile dysfunction
  - Decreased libido
  - Premature ejaculation
- This chapter will evaluate the different pharmaceutical regimens for the above conditions.
- As always, a thorough history and physical examination (including psychological history affecting sexual function) is critical.

■ Erectile Dysfunction

- Erectile dysfunction is defined by the National Institutes of Health as an erection insufficient for sexual function.[1]
- Medical optimization of systemic comorbidities should be controlled and/or eliminated. These include:
  - Hypertension
  - Diabetes mellitus
  - Depression
  - Hyperlipidemia
  - Alcoholism
  - Smoking
- Other medications can have a detrimental effect on libido and/or achieving a satisfactory erection. These include:
  - Benzodiazepines
  - Antidepressants (TCA, SSRI)
  - Metaclopremide
  - Marijuana
  - Antihypertensives (alpha/beta-blockers and thiazides)

- First-line therapy should include phosphodiesterase (PDE-5) inhibitors, unless contraindicated. There has been no consensus about which is best, sildenafil, vardenafil, or tadalafil.

Sildenafil (Viagra)

- Administer 25–100 mg PO one hour before sexual stimulation; effects last four hours.
- This was the first drug approved for treatment of erectile dysfunction.
- Goldstein compared the effects of sildenafil to that of a placebo in people with varying forms of erectile dysfunction (organic, psychogenic, or mixed). He discovered that sexual intercourse was achievable in 69% of patients taking sildenafil as compared to placebo.[2]
- 10 tablets of 100 mg cost $155.99.*

Vardenafil (Levitra)

- Administer 5–20mg PO one hour before sexual stimulation; effects last four hours.
- Hellstrom, and colleagues found vardenafil to be as effective as sildenafil at successfully overcoming erectile dysfunction as per the International Index of Erectile Function.
  - It should be noted that in this study, vardenafil was not compared directly to sildenafil.
  - This was a double-blind, 26-week placebo-controlled study.[3]
  - Success was defined as achieving penetration and maintaining an erection.
- 10 tablets of 20 mg cost $153.99.*

Tadalafil (Cialis)

- Administer 5–20 mg PO before sexual stimulation (effects last 12 to 36 hours) or 2.5–5 mg PO per day.
- This drug is not affected by alcohol.

---

*Prices quoted from drugstore.com

- Brock et al. evaluated 1112 patients with an average age of 59 years who were assigned to either placebo or tadalafil groups (daily doses of 2.5 mg, 5 mg, 10 mg, or 20 mg).
  - Patients receiving 20 mg a day of tadalafil noted 81% improvement in erections, compared to 35% in the control group.[4]
- 10 tablets of 20 mg cost $171.99.*
- A recent meta-analysis completed by Tsertsvadze and associates indicated that all three phosphodiesterase inhibitors were beneficial at increasing success of sexual intercourse when compared to placebo (69% to 35%).[5]
- The most common adverse effect of the above medications has been reported to be headache, with between 8 and 18% of patients reporting this effect, followed by flushing, reported by 6–13%. This is because all three medications cause peripheral dilation. Other reported side effects include dyspepsia and altered vision.[6]
- Do not use any of the PDE-5 inhibitors if the patient:
  - Is taking nitrates
  - Has a prior heart history (without medical clearance from cardiology)
  - Has QT prolongation (as with vardenafil).
- Care should be taken to hepatically dose those with liver dysfunction will all three PDE-5 medications.
- If a patient fails treatment with one particular PDE-5, it is reasonable to attempt treatment with another PDE-5. If the second attempt fails to produce adequate results, progress to other treatments (as outlined as follows).

Yohimbine (Aphrodyne)

- This medication originates from the yohimbe tree.
- It is often a component in male enhancement medications.
- It works as an alpha 2–adrenergic inhibitor.

*Prices quoted from drugstore.com

- It is not recommended in the 2005 American Urological Association guidelines for the treatment of erectile dysfunction.
  - Weiner associated yohimbine with such adverse effects as:
    - Increased blood pressure
    - Increased heart rate
    - Irritability[7]
  - Kunelius failed to show an improvement in erectile dysfunction when compared to placebo.[8]

Vacuum Erection Device (VED)

- This device is used in conjunction with an occlusive ring at the base of the penis.
- A cylindrical pump is applied to the penis, causing a "vacuum" effect of blood flowing to the penis. The occlusive ring is then applied to maintain the erection.
- A study conducted in Singapore by Tay and Kim evaluated VED with 18 men using questionnaires over a six-month period,
  - After one week, 13 patients (72.2%) reported being confident in using the device, and 88.9% of patients reported achieving satisfactory erections.[9]
- There have been publications of unique complications with this method:
  - Urethral bleeding
  - Capture of scrotal tunica within the penile shaft
  - Cystic mass formation
  - Peyronie's disease
  - All patients who reported these effects ceased using VED after treatment for the aforementioned effects.[10]
- One of the larger studies on VED was performed by Opsomer et al., who studied VED in 110 patients between the ages of 36 and 75 over a three-year period.[11]

Medicated Urethral System for Erection (MUSE)

- This is a special form of Alprostadil that is inserted into the urethra.

- It promotes erectile function by increasing the concentration of cAMP, which decreases intracellular calcium, resulting in erection due to relaxation of smooth muscle and dilation of cavernosal arteries.
- Contraindications to its use include, but are not limited to:
  - Peyronie's disease
  - Balanitis
  - Urethritis
  - Stricture
- Guay et al. studied 277 patients who were administered dosages of Alprostadil between 500 micrograms and 1000 micrograms.
  - In this study, 56% of patients reported having satisfactory completion of sexual intercourse in more than 66% of attempts.[12]
- Padma-Nathan and colleagues used MUSE in a double-blind, placebo-controlled study of 1511 patients.
  - Each patient was instructed in the correct application in office and then was assigned 125, 250, 500, or 1000 micrograms per day of either Alprostadil or placebo for three months at home.
  - Researchers reported the efficacy of this drug in achieving erections sufficient for intercourse in 64.9%, compared to 18.6% in placebo, with painful erections being the most reported side effect.
  - Of the men who responded to the treatment, 70% were able to engage in sexual intercourse.[13]
- After administration of the medication, it is important to instruct the patient to massage his penis to make sure the medication is distributed throughout the cavernosal bodies.
- Also instruct the patient not to use more than two applications per 24 hours (with a maximal dose of 1000 micrograms).
- Inform the patient that he may experience:
  - Burning
  - Bleeding

- Priapism
- Hypotension
- Potential other side effects

Intracavernosal Injections

- This is the most effective nonsurgical treatment of erectile dysfunction.
- There are three possible medications that can be injected intracavernosally:
  - Papaverine (PDE inhibitor)
  - Phentolamine (alpha-adrenergic receptor inhibitor, needs to be used in conjunction with either papaverine or alprostadil because its function is to prevent detumescence and not to cause an erection in itself)
  - Alprostadil (function is to increase cAMP)
- The first administration should be performed by the urologist in order to educate the patient and to determine the efficacy of the treatment.
- Each of the above medications carries with it the risk of certain adverse effects.
  - When alprostadil is compared to papaverine, alprostadil shows lower rates of priapism and penile fibrosis.
  - Kulmala and Tamella believe that erections lasting longer than 36 hours should be treated with puncture and administration of alpha-adrenergic drugs. If present for longer than 48 hours, a shunt is needed.[14]
    - In the men who required shunts, fibrosis of the cavernosal muscle was the end result (no fibrosis was seen in erections lasting less than 36 hours).
    - However, the majority of patients could continue to use the intracavernosal injection after successful treatment of the priapism.

Trazadone

- Trazadone was hypothesized by Fink et al. to improve erectile dysfunction by inhibiting alpha 2–adrenergic receptors, leading to enhanced arterial flow.
- However, no benefit was shown when compared to placebo.[15]

According to the American Urological Association update by Montague et al., this drug should not be used for the treatment of erectile dysfunction.[16]

Decreased Libido

- "Loss of libido refers to reduction in sexual interest, initiative, frequency and intensity of responses to internal or external erotic stimuli . . . factors include psychogenic, CNS disease, androgen deficiency and resistance, and side effects from medications."[17]
- Common medications/agents producing these effects are alcohol, blood pressure medications, and psychotropics.
- The differential diagnosis for decreased libido should include chronic fatigue syndrome, hypogonadism, hypothryoidism, and psychological conditions.[18]
- Morning testosterone is used for evaluation of sexual dysfunction. If testosterone is low, further work-up should entail FSH, LH, prolactin, and a repeat testosterone.
- The goals of testosterone replacement therapy include:
  - Restoring normal sexual function and sexual drive
  - Optimizing bone density
  - Prevention of osteoporosis
  - Improving energy and well-being
  - Improving mood and cognition
  - Improving fertility in those with hypogonadotrophic hypogonadism
  - Possible reduction in the risk of cardiovascular disease
- There are various testosterone formulations available for use and include: intramuscular injections, subcutaneous implants, and topical agents.
- Intramuscular injectible agents can be self-administered and often dosed weekly or biweekly. Their disadvantages include the need for a deep intramuscular injection of a large volume of material. Serum testosterone levels may fluctuate and, thus, symptoms may wax and wane.
- Subcutaneous injections can be in a pellet form and have the advantage of having a long duration of action (up to six months). Disadvantages include the need for a minor

surgical procedure for implantation, infection and extrusion of the pellets.

- Topical agents can include topical gels, transdermal patches that can be placed on the skin of the scrotum, non scrotal skin or in the buccal mucosa.
  - Topical gels are well tolerated and easy to use. However, they must be applied daily. There is potential for the gel to rub off, which may limit efficacy, and they can be expensive.
  - Transdermal patches can be applied to the scrotum or nonscrotal skin. These are easy to apply. Side effects include skin irritation and can be expensive.
  - Buccal mucosal systems are also available and considered to be a form of transdermal testosterone. Side effects include mouth and gum irritation as well as alteration of taste. These may require twice daily application for best efficacy. It is possible to swallow the small patch. This therapy can be cost limiting in some.
- Rhoden and Morgentaler looked at testosterone replacement therapy in hypogonadal men at high risk for prostate cancer. In a study of 75 hypogonadal men that were followed for 12 months with testosterone replacement with prostate biopsies prior were found not to have a greater increase in PSA or significant increase risk of developing prostate cancer.[19]

Premature Ejaculation

- The 2004 AUA guidelines reports that premature ejaculation is "ejaculation that occurs sooner than desired, either before or shortly after penetration, causing distress to either one or both partners."[20] History and physical is always important but obtaining information from the partner is imperative.
- Premature ejaculation can be a lifelong problem that is characterized by ejaculation that occurs too early at nearly every intercourse with nearly every woman. Most males with this condition ejaculate within 60 seconds of penetration.
- Acquired premature ejaculation implies that the individual had normal ejaculation prior to the start of his

complaints. This condition may be due to an underlying physical problem such as ED, prostatitis, thyroid dysfunction or an underlying psychologic disturbance. This condition may be assuaged by treatment of the underlying cause. For example, treatment of the patient with prostatitis who has premature ejaculation may be helped by treatment of the prostatitis with antibiotics and anti-inflammatory agents.

- Natural variable premature ejaculation can occur coincidentally and/or situationally. This may be due to a normal variation in the male sexual response cycle. Patients complain of early ejaculations that are inconsistent and irregular with interspersed normal sexual intercourse.

- Premature-like ejaculatory dysfunction is usually not due to an underlying medical reason. Patients subjectively perceive rapid ejaculation and become preoccupied by this. These patients likely have a normal intravaginal ejaculatory latency time of between 5 and 25 minutes.

- Often times there is a combination of premature ejaculation and erectile dysfunction, in those circumstances the physician should try and correct the erectile dysfunction first. After this, antidepressants are often the treatment of choice, SSRIs (Fluoxetine [5–20 mg daily], Paroxetine [10–40 mg daily], Sertraline [25–200 mg daily]), or Clomipramine (25–50 mg daily). If the patient wished not to take a daily antidepressant, the previous medications could be taken, on average, four hours prior to intercourse to achieve the desired effect. In a double-blind, randomized, placebo-controlled study with fluoxetine, fluvoxamine, paroxetine, and Sertraline, intravaginal ejaculation latency time increased on average from 20 seconds to 110 seconds, with the best results using Paroxetine. The results were conducted through surveys in approximately 60 men over a six week period.[21]

■ Conclusions

- There are several oral agents used to treat erectile dysfunction. Each has been shown to be effective versus placebo in controlled trials. The agents appear to be similarly effective in the treatment of ED.

- The Vacuum Erection Device, Intracavernosal injection agents, and MUSE are considered to be second line agents in the treatment of ED.

- It is important to recognize low libido states and premature ejaculation and differentiate these conditions from erectile dysfunction. The treatment of these conditions, as shown in this chapter, are different from the treatment of ED.

- Finally, it is important to consider that ED, premature ejaculation and low libido states may occur in the same patient. Thus, treatment may involve several treatments in selected patients.

■ References

1. Impotence. NIH consensus statement. 1992;10:1.

2. Goldstein I, Lue TF, Padma-Nathan H, Rosen RC, Steers WD, Wicker PA. Oral sildenafil in the treatment of erectile dysfunction. *N Engl J Med.* 1998;338:1997.

3. Hellstrom W, Gittelman M, Karlin G, et al. Sustained efficacy and tolerability of vardenafil, a highly potent selective phosphodiesterase type 5 inhibitor, in men with erectile dysfunction: results of a randomized, double-blind, 26-week placebo-controlled pivotal trial. *Urology.* 2004;61:8–14.

4. Brock G, McMahon C, Point P, et al. Efficacy and safety of tadalafil for the treatment of erectile dysfunction: result of integrated analyses. *J Urol.* 2005;173:664.

5. Tsertsvadze A, Fink H, Yazdi F, et al. Oral phosphodiesterase-5 inhibitors and hormonal treatments for erectile dysfunction: a systematic review and meta-analysis. *Ann Intern Med.* 2009;151(9):650–661.

6. Ellsworth P, Kirshenbaum E. Current concepts in the evaluation and management of erectile dysfunction. *Urol Nurs.* 2008;28:357–369.

7. Weiner N. Drugs that inhibit adrenergic nerves and block adrenergic receptors. In: Gilman AG, Goodman LS, Rall TW, Murad F, eds. *Goodman and Gilman's The Pharmacological Basis of Therapeutics,* 7th ed. New York, NY: MacMillan; 1985:181–214

8. Kunelius P, Hakkinen J, Lukkarinen O. Is high-dose yohim-
    bine hydrochloride effective in the treatment of mixed-type
    impotence? A prospective, randomized, controlled double-
    blind crossover study. *Urology*. 1997;49:441.

9. Tay K, Lim P. A prospective trial with vacuum-assisted erec-
    tion devices. *Ann Acad Med Singapore*. 1997;24:705–707.

10. Ganem J, Lucey D, Janosko E, Carson C. Unusual com-
    plications of the vacuum erection device. *Urology*.
    1998;51(4):627–631.

11. Opsomer R, Wese F, De Groote P, Van Cangh P. The exter-
    nal vacuum device in the management of erectile dysfunc-
    tion. *Acta Urol Belg*. 1997;65:13–16.

12. Guay AT, Perez JB, Velasquez E, Newton RA, Jacobson JP.
    Clinical experience with intraurethral alprostadil (MUSE)
    in the treatment of men with erectile dysfunction. A ret-
    rospective study. Medicated Urethral System for Erection.
    Eur Urol. 2000;38:671–676.

13. Padma-Nathan H, Hellstrom WJ, Kaiser F, et al. Treatment
    of men with erectile dysfunction with transurethral alprosta-
    dil. Medicated Urethral System for Erection (MUSE) Study
    Group. *N Engl J Med*. 1997;336:1–7.

14. Kumala R, Tamella T. Effects of priapism lasting 24 hours
    or longer caused by intracavernosal injection of vasoactive
    drugs. *Int J Impot Res*. 1995;7:131.

15. Fink HA, MacDonald R, Rutks, IR, and Wilt TJ. Trazadone
    for erectile dysfunction: a systematic review and metaanaly-
    sis. *Br J Urol*. 2006;92:441.

16. Montague D, Jarrow JP, Broderick GA, Dmochowski
    RR, Heaton JP, Lue TF, et al. Chapter 1: the manage-
    ment of erectile dysfunction: an AUA update. *J Urol*.
    2005;174:230–239.

17. Swerdloff RS, Wang C. The testis and male sexual function.
    In: Goldman L, Ausiello D, eds. *Cecil Medicine*, 23rd ed.
    Philadelphia, Pa: Saunders Elsevier; 2007:chap 252.

18. Heidelbaugh JJ. Management of erectile dysfunction. *Am
    Fam Physician*. 2010;81:305–312.

19. Rhoden EL, Morgentaler A. Testosterone replacement
    therapy in hypogonadal men at high risk for prostate cancer:
    results of 1 year of treatment in men with prostate intraepi-
    thelial neoplasia. *J Urol*. 2003;170:2348–2351.

20. Montague K, Jarrow J, Broderick GA, et al. AUA guidelines
    on the pharmacologic management of premature ejacula-
    tion. *J Urol*. 2004;172(1):290–294.

21.   Waldinger MD, Hengeveld MW, Zwinderman AH, <u>Olivier</u>
      B. Effect of SSI antidepressants on ejaculation: a double-
      blind, randomized, placebo-controlled study with fluox-
      etine, fluvoxamine, paroxetine, and sertraline. *J Clin
      Psychopharmacol.* 2001;21:241–242.

CHAPTER 5

Surgical Treatment for Erectile Dysfunction

Aimee E. Rogers, MD ■ *Stanley Zaslau, MD, MBA, FACS*

■ Introduction

- Erectile dysfunction affects approximately 300,000 to 400,000 American men each year.[1]
- The prevalence of erectile dysfunction increases with age.
  - Of men aged 40 and older, 52% have some degree of erectile dysfunction.[2]
- Most men with erectile dysfunction are initially offered systemic therapy with a phosphodiesterase type 5 (PDE-5) inhibitor, such as sildenafil (Viagra). When systemic therapy fails, and the man wishes to continue treatment, second- and third-line therapies, such as vacuum erection devices and intracavernosal injections, are usually considered.
- Surgical intervention still has a clear role in the management of patients with erectile dysfunction when both the systemic and other approaches fail or are contraindicated.
- The surgical treatments of erectile dysfunction will be reviewed in this chapter. These include:
  - Penile revascularization surgery
  - Venous ligation
  - Penile prostheses
- Correction of penile curvature, as well as other aspects of erectile dysfunction, will be discussed separately.

■ Penile Prostheses

History

- The use of penile prostheses for the treatment of erectile dysfunction began in the 1950s.
  - The first implants consisted of rib cartilage, modeled after the penis of some animals.[3]

- As technology advanced, other materials were placed subcutaneously, such as:
  - Polyethylene rods
  - Acrylic splints
  - Pure silicone implants
- A major advance in penile prosthetic surgery was the insertion of these devices into the paired corpora cavernosa, which provided greater cosmetic and functional results.[4]
- During the early years of penile prosthetic implantation, most of these devices were plagued by mechanical failure that usually required revision or removal.
- Today, penile prostheses have become reliable mechanical devices associated with a relatively high level of patient satisfaction.[5]

Malleable versus Inflatable Prostheses

- There are currently four types of penile prostheses available to men in the United States:
  - The semirigid rod
  - The positional prosthesis
  - The two-piece inflatable prosthesis
  - The three-piece inflatable prosthesis.
- These four types of prostheses belong to two principal categories of penile prostheses: the inflatable and the malleable, or semirigid, devices.
  - Inflatable devices are selected most often by patients because they mimic a normally functioning penis in that they are able to achieve both rigidity and flaccidity.
  - Insertion of a malleable prosthesis, on the other hand, results in a "permanent" erection that is bent up or down, depending on the situation and the needs of the patient.
  - Malleable, or semirigid, devices make up less than 10% of all implanted penile prostheses and are typically used by patients with less manual dexterity because of their ease of use.[6]

Patient Considerations

- Several factors determine which type of implant to use in a given patient.
- The first factor to consider is the mental and manual dexterity of the patient.
  - Older men, especially those with limited mental and/or manual dexterity, are usually better served by a malleable prosthesis. This is because it may be too challenging or cumbersome for these men to manipulate the pump and deflation mechanisms in the inflatable devices.[7]
- Patients with injuries to the spinal cord that result in diminished sensation in the penis may be better served by an inflatable device.
  - This is due to the risk of prolonged excessive pressure that the firm prosthetic rods of a malleable device would exert on the penile tissues, resulting in erosion of the rods through the skin or urethra.[8]
- In general, most men with adequate mental function and manual dexterity choose the inflatable penile prosthesis because they prefer its capability to mimic the normal penis, both for its usual state of flaccidity and for its ability to become rigid for sexual activity.[9]

Types of Prostheses

Malleable or Semirigid Prosthesis

- Malleable penile prostheses are semirigid devices with a central core that allows the penis to be bent down when not in use and bent upward for sexual activity.[10]
- They have been available for several decades.
- When a malleable prosthesis is implanted, a permanent erection occurs.
  - However, the prosthetic device can be bent down close to the body and can be relatively well concealed under clothing.
  - When sexual activity is anticipated, the penis is simply bent upward.
- Malleable prostheses bend with relative ease, but they do have a springback phenomenon. They have some

"memory" as to their original shape and ultimately return to some degree to their original straight position.[11]

- Malleable devices have the advantage of very low mechanical failure rates and ease of use. Disadvantages include constant penile rigidity and an increased risk of erosion.[12]

Positional Prosthesis

- The positional penile prosthesis (Dura II, American Medical Systems Inc., Minnetonka, MN) is similar to the malleable prosthesis in that it is also a semirigid device.
- However, unlike the malleable device, the positional penile prosthesis has a central series of articulating segments held together with a spring on each end. This device is therefore better able to maintain its upward and downward positions, and thus has less of a springback phenomenon.[13]
- The advantages and disadvantages of this device are similar to that of the malleable semirigid prosthesis.

Two-Piece Inflatable Prosthesis

- The two-piece penile prosthesis is one of the two inflatable devices offered to men with erectile dysfunction.
- It consists of two cylinders connected to a small scrotal pump.
- Inflation of the device is achieved by squeezing the scrotal pump, which redistributes fluid from the rear tip reservoirs of the cylinders into a nondistensible central chamber in the front of the cylinders.
  - This creates rigidity in the outward aspect of the corpora cavernosa, thus creating an erection.
- Deflation is accomplished by bending the cylinders within the penis, which activates a valve that allows the fluid to return to the reservoir area at the base of the cylinders.[14]
- The main advantage of the two-piece penile prosthesis is that there is no need for a separate reservoir, which makes implantation easier than that of the three-piece prosthesis.

- The device also comes complete and requires no filling or connections intra-operatively.
- The two-piece implant is well suited for men who have had prior pelvic or inguinal surgery, in whom surgical placement of a separate reservoir may be more problematic.
- The two-piece device also requires less dexterity and digital sensitivity than do other multicomponent devices.
- On the other hand, the two-piece prosthesis appears fuller than the three-piece device in the flaccid state because less fluid can be transferred to the smaller reservoir area.[15]
- A disadvantage compared with the malleable devices is the increased risk of mechanical failure.

Three-Piece Inflatable Prosthesis

- The ideal prosthesis would provide its recipient with a penis that mimics as closely as possible normal penile flaccidity and erection. Only three-piece inflatable devices that transfer a large volume of fluid into the penile cylinders for erection and out of the cylinders for flaccidity approach this ideal.[16]
- Three-piece prostheses consist of:
  - Paired corporeal cylinders
  - A scrotal pump/deflation mechanism
  - An abdominal fluid reservoir
- Erection is achieved by repeatedly squeezing the pump located within the scrotum.
  - Each compression transfers fluid from the reservoir to the intracorporeal cylinders until adequate pressure is achieved, thus creating an erection.
- Deflation is achieved by pressing a valve mechanism located next to the scrotal pump, permitting fluid to flow out of the cylinders and return to the reservoir.[17]
- Both the two-piece and three-piece penile prostheses are designed to approximate the rigidity and flaccidity of the normally functioning penis.
- With these devices, two hollow cylinders are placed within the corpora cavernosa, a fluid reservoir is placed

behind the pubic bone, and a pump is situated in the scrotum.

- Rear tip extenders can be added to the back of the cylinders to modify penile length further.[18]

■ All three-piece devices provide penile girth expansion and rigidity similar to that of a normal erection. One device, the AMS 700 Ultrex (American Medical Systems Inc., Minnetonka, MN), also provides length expansion.[19]

■ The advantages of three-piece devices are similar to those of the two-piece device: They mimic a normally functioning penis and pose less risk of erosion.

■ The main disadvantages of three-piece penile prostheses are the increased risk of mechanical failure and the relative complexity of its insertion. Furthermore, the three-piece device does require relative mental and manual dexterity on the part of the patient for its successful use.[20]

Preoperative Considerations

■ Discussions regarding the treatment of erectile dysfunction ideally should include the patient's partner, but this is not always possible.

■ Penile prosthesis implantation should not be considered to treat a man with erectile dysfunction that is situational, the result of a relationship conflict, or potentially reversible.

- For these men and their partners, psychological consultation and sex therapy are more appropriate.

■ Once a decision has been made regarding insertion of a penile prosthesis, the various types of penile prostheses along with their advantages and disadvantages should be discussed.

■ It is important for the patient to understand that penile prostheses produce an erectionlike state. The glans penis is not included in an erection achieved using a prosthesis, and for most men the length of their erect penis is shorter than their normal erection.

■ Many men with erectile dysfunction have normal libido, and most have normal penile sensation and orgasm with ejaculation. Penile prosthesis implantation preserves orgasm and ejaculation if present, but does not restore them if they are absent.[21]

Preoperative Preparation

- Prior to the procedure, the patient should be informed of the various risks and benefits of the procedure. This includes the risk of:
  - Infection
  - Erosion
  - Bleeding
  - Mechanical failure
- The patient should be informed that infection would likely result in complete explantation of the implant, with resulting scarring of the bilateral corpora.
- He should also understand that mechanical failure is possible and correcting it requires device revision or replacement.[22]
- Preoperative preparation of the prosthesis recipient is directed primarily at reducing the risk of infection.
  - The recipient should be free of urinary tract infection.
  - He should have no infections elsewhere that might result in bacterial seeding during the healing phase.[23]
  - While better control of diabetes mellitus may reduce risk of infection, the literature fails to demonstrate a consistent benefit.[24]
  - There should be no other wounds, dermatitis, or other breaks in the skin in the operative field.

Procedure

- The procedure is performed with the patient in the supine position under either spinal or general anesthesia.
- The operative area is shaved immediately prior to the first incision to avoid bacterial colonization of small skin breaks that might occur if shaving is performed by the patient prior to the procedure.
- After the patient is shaved, a thorough 10-minute skin preparation is performed.[25]
- Broad-spectrum intravenous antibiotics providing both gram-positive and gram-negative coverage are administered

prophylactically before the initial incision is made and may be continued for 24 to 48 hours postoperatively.[26]

- Frequently used antibiotics for gram-positive coverage include ampicillin, vancomycin, or the cephalosporins. For gram-negative coverage, aminoglycosides or fluoroquinolones are suggested.

■ Placement of the prosthetic device can be performed through a penoscrotal, infrapubic, or subcoronal approach.

- The subcoronal approach is used only for implantation of malleable or positional devices.

■ A 4-cm transverse incision is made about one centimeter below the penoscrotal junction. This incision is dissected down to the level of the dartos fascia, toward the urethra and the corporal bodies.

■ The underside of the dartos fascia is dissected away from the urethra and the proximal portion of the corpora, or crura.

■ Corporotomies of 2 cm are made, and two horizontal mattress sutures are placed on each side.

- These sutures are used as guides during corporeal dilation and measurement, and are ultimately used to close each corporotomy after the cylinders are placed.

■ Dilation of the corpora then begins with an 8-mm dilator and proceeds to 16 mm proximally and to 14 mm distally. The proximal portion is dilated to a greater extent to accommodate both the cylinder and the cylinder tubing.

■ Following dilation, both proximal and distal measurements are taken from their respective ends of the corporotomy.

■ After corporeal measurements are taken, the appropriate cylinder size is chosen, both in terms of length and diameter.

■ Both cylinders are then inserted into the bilateral corpora with the use of a cylinder inserter.

■ Rear tip extenders are added to the ends of the cylinders as needed.

■ Both corporotomies are then closed by tying the proximal and distal ends of the preplaced horizontal mattress sutures.[27]

- The pump is placed in the scrotum via a second incision made through the dartos fascia in the scrotal septum.
- If a three-piece implant is chosen, a separate reservoir is placed into the retropubic space through the primary penoscrotal incision via the external inguinal ring, or through a separate lower abdominal incision.
- The operation may be performed as an outpatient procedure.
- The patient is instructed to avoid using the device for four to six weeks to allow for adequate healing.[28]

Postoperative Care

- A urethral catheter is maintained to gravity drainage until the following morning.
- Oral antibiotic therapy is usually continued for one week after discharge.
- Oral narcotics are usually required for about a week after surgery.
- If a reservoir has been placed, the patient is instructed to avoid lifting and other activities that might result in reservoir displacement.
- Approximately one month after surgery, most men are ready to learn how to operate the device.
  - The patient is instructed to inflate the device using the pump located within the scrotum.
  - He then can deflate the device by applying pressure to the deflation mechanism, also located within the scrotum.
- The patient practices 'cycling' the device twice daily for approximately one month.
- After a month, the patient is given permission to use the device for sexual intercourse whenever inflation can be accomplished with ease and without discomfort.[29]

Complications

- The patient considering penile prosthesis implantation should be made aware of the potential complications of the procedure, including:
  - Infection
  - Erosion

- Mechanical failure and resulting reoperation
- Penile shortening
- Urethral injury
- Impaired sensation[30]

Infection

- The most serious complication of penile prosthesis implantation is infection.
- According to Jarow and colleagues, infection occurs in approximately 3% of cases, and in up to 10% of higher-risk cases, such as in men with diabetes, spinal cord injury, or prior implants.[31]
- Causative organisms are usually skin flora, in particular, staphylococcus species such as *staphylococcus epidermidis*, suggesting that bacterial seeding occurs at the time of implantation.[32]
- Early infections are usually indicated by the presence of:
  - Swelling
  - Erythema
  - Tenderness over the affected area
  - Possible purulent drainage
  - Occasionally fever
- Late infections are usually manifested only by persistent or recurrent long-term pain in the area of the implant.
  - With long-term infections, the scrotal skin has been found to be adherent to the pump.[33]
- Treatment of the prosthetic infection with intravenous antibiotics usually results in clinical improvement, but the antibiotic treatment rarely permanently eradicates this type of infection.
  - According to Abouassaly and colleagues, this is thought to be due to harboring of microorganisms within a biofilm that is adherent to the device.[34]
  - For this reason, when a prosthesis is infected, all components of the device should be removed.
  - Therefore, infection is considered by many to be the most significant complication of genitourinary prosthetic surgery.[35]
- In the past, a majority of the penile prostheses that were removed due to infection were not considered

for reimplantation during the same procedure. Reimplantation was often delayed as long as a year.

- During this time, the scar within the corpora would mature, resulting in contraction, which resulted in a smaller penis size and more difficulty with dilation after cylinder reimplantation.
- Reimplantation at that time was therefore more difficult to perform successfully.
- However, pump and reservoir reimplantation was and still is seldom a problem.
  - To minimize loss of penile size and to facilitate corporeal dilation, many experts now perform prosthesis reimplantation as soon as possible after device removal for infection.
  - Reimplantation is usually performed approximately two to three months after device removal, when all the incisions have healed and postoperative edema has resolved.[36]
- Mulcahy and colleagues first introduced the concept of prosthesis salvage for infection.
  - Their protocol involves removal of all prosthetic components and foreign bodies, followed by copious irrigation with seven antibacterial solutions.
  - A new device is implanted thereafter.
  - Of 55 patients reimplanted in this fashion, 45 (82%) were free of infection, with follow-up ranging from 6 to 93 months.[37]
  - When salvage procedures are successful, they maintain penile length and rectify the problem with only one operation.
  - If the entire device is explanted and all prosthesis compartments are copiously irrigated before a new prosthesis is implanted, the infection rate is not significantly different from the rates seen with first-time prosthesis implantation.[38]

Erosion

- Erosion of a penile prosthesis is uncommon.
- The most common sites of erosion are the distal cylinder and the scrotal pump. The likely reasons for these

sites as areas to erode are the lack of distal penile sensation in the patient with a spinal cord injury, diabetes, or someone who has previously undergone external beam irradiation.

- Erosion is also possible if an oversized prosthesis is used. This can lead to erosion by tissue pressure atrophy and necrosis.
- Erosion can also occur if a patient keeps the prosthesis inflated when they are not using it. This can also lead to tissue pressure atrophy and necrosis.
- Erosion of the reservoir into the bladder or into the bowel are extremely rare complications.
- The scrotally placed penile implant pump can also erode. This can occur in patients with impaired sensation such as diabetics and patients with spinal cord injury.

Mechanical Failure and Subsequent Operation

- True mechanical failures for inflatable penile prostheses include leakage of fluid from various points including:
  - Tubing leak
  - Pump leak
  - Reservoir leak
  - Cylinder aneurysm
- While individual components may be at fault, it is the author's recommendation that the individual component be replaced if the implant was initially placed in the preceding 12 months. If the implant has been in place for longer that 12 months, the entire device should be replaced.

Penile Shortening

- Penile shortening is likely to occur after placement of a penile prosthesis. This can be due to ischemia of corporal and tunica albiginea layers of the corpus cavernosa. This is common in patients with ED of many years duration.
- It is important to counsel patients preoperatively about the likelihood of penile shortening after penile prosthesis implantation. This will improve patient satisfaction postoperatively.

- It is possible to perform a ligation of the penile suspensory ligament in an effort to gain additional penile length. In the author's opinion, while this may produce additional penile length, the penis is more floppy and can hang lower because of its lack of ligamentous support.

Urethral Injury

- Urethral injury can occur during dilation of the corporal bodies during placement of the prosthesis.
- This injury is likely to be more common in patients who have had prior pelvic external beam irradiation, have diabetes mellitus, or who have suffered a pelvic fracture.
- Care must be taken not to injure the urethra during the procedure. For distal urethral injuries, the implant procedure should be abandoned and the patient left with a urinary catheter in place. A second procedure can be undertaken after three months. For proximal urethral injuries, the urethral injury can be repaired over a urinary catheter. While one could consider placement of the penile implant at this time, the authors recommend waiting until the urethral injury has healed and then undertake a second operation at a later date.

Impaired Sensation

- Patients who are diabetics, have a history of spinal cord injury, or have received pelvic irradiation are at increased risk for loss of penile sensation after placement of a penile implant.
- It is likely that the patient's underlying disease state resulted in the impaired penile sensation rather than the implant procedure causing this complication.
- In such patients, malleable penile implants are more likely to cause erosion particularly because the patient will not feel the implant. In fact, such patients may not realized that erosion has occurred until there is secondary infection present. These patients are better served with a three-piece inflatable prosthesis because it can be deflated, which can minimize the risk of erosion.

■ Vascular Surgery for Erectile Dysfunction

History

- The first cases of penile arterial bypass surgery for erectile dysfunction were reported by Michal and colleagues in the early 1970s, using the inferior epigastric artery as the donor vessel.[39]

- Subsequent modifications by Virag and others resulted in a multitude of procedures that used the deep dorsal vein as the recipient vessel.[40]

- Crespo and colleagues presented procedures for revascularization of the cavernosal artery directly by use of the inferior epigastric artery as a donor source.[41]

- Lack of standardized techniques and selection criteria may contribute to the current low popularity of arterial revascularization. To date, no single procedure has been universally accepted.

Indications

- Vascular surgical procedures, particularly penile arterial revascularization and penile venous surgery, are recommended only for a select group of patients.

- Several series have reported reasonable success for penile arterial reconstructive surgery if performed in young, nonsmoking, healthy men with recently acquired erectile dysfunction secondary to focal arterial occlusion with no evidence of generalized vascular disease.[42]

- According to DePalma and colleagues, only 6–7% of men with vascular erectile dysfunction are candidates for arterial reconstructive surgery.[43]

- Another study performed years later revealed that success rates in older men with diabetes or other evidence of generalized vascular disease were also very low.[44]

■ Conclusions

- Surgical intervention has an important role in the management of patients with ED when systemic and other approaches fail or are contraindicated.

- Physicians must always consider the mental and manual dexterity of the patient when selecting a malleable versus inflatable prosthesis.
- Physicians must carefully explain to patients and their partners the risks and benefits of penile implant surgery before performing any procedure.

■ References

1. Lue TF. Erectile dysfunction. *N Engl J Med*. 2000;342: 1802.
2. Broderick GA, Lue TF. Evaluation and nonsurgical management of erectile dysfunction and premature ejaculation. In: Wein AJ, Kavoussi LR, Novick AC, Partin AW, Peters CA, eds. *Campbell-Walsh Urology*. 9th ed. Philadelphia, PA: Saunders Elsevier Company; 2007:750–787.
3. Morgentaler A. Male impotence. *Lancet*. 1999;354:1713.
4. Scott FB, Bradley WE, Timm GW. Management of erectile impotence: use of implantable penile prostheses. *Urology*. 1973;2:80.
5. Lazarou S. Surgical treatment of erectile dysfunction. *UpToDate*. 2009.
6. Wilson S. Penile prostheses at the millennium. *Contemp Urol*. 2001;35.
7. Lazarou S. Surgical treatment of erectile dysfunction. *UpToDate*. 2009.
8. Gross AJ, Sauerwein DH, Kutzenberger J, Ringert RH. Penile prostheses in paraplegic men. *Br J Urology*. 1996;78: 262.
9. Lazarou S. Surgical treatment of erectile dysfunction. *UpToDate*. 2009.
10. Montague DK. Prosthetic surgery for erectile dysfunction. In: Wein AJ, Kavoussi LR, Novick AC, Partin AW, Peters CA, eds. *Campbell-Walsh Urology*. 9th ed. Philadelphia, PA: Saunders Elsevier Company; 2007:788–801.
11. Lazarou S. Surgical treatment of erectile dysfunction. *UpToDate*. 2009.
12. Montague DK. Prosthetic surgery for erectile dysfunction. In: Wein AJ, Kavoussi LR, Novick AC, Partin AW, Peters CA, eds. *Campbell-Walsh Urology*. 9th ed. Philadelphia, PA: Saunders Elsevier Company; 2007:788–801.
13. Montague DK. Prosthetic surgery for erectile dysfunction. In: Wein AJ, Kavoussi LR, Novick AC, Partin AW, Peters CA, eds. *Campbell-Walsh Urology*. 9th ed. Philadelphia, PA: Saunders Elsevier Company; 2007:788–801.

14. Lazarou S. Surgical treatment of erectile dysfunction. *UpToDate*. 2009.

15. Khoudary KP, Morgentaler A. Design considerations in penile prostheses: the American Medical Systems product line. *J Long Term Eff Med Implants*. 1997;7:55.

16. Montague DK. Prosthetic surgery for erectile dysfunction. In: Wein AJ, Kavoussi LR, Novick AC, Partin AW, Peters CA, eds. *Campbell-Walsh Urology*. 9th ed. Philadelphia, PA: Saunders Elsevier Company; 2007:788–801.

17. Lazarou S. Surgical treatment of erectile dysfunction. *UpToDate*. 2009.

18. Quesada ET, Light JK. The AMS 700 inflatable penile prosthesis: long-term experience with the controlled expansion cylinder. *J Urol*. 1993;149:46.

19. Montague DK. Prosthetic surgery for erectile dysfunction. In: Wein AJ, Kavoussi LR, Novick AC, Partin AW, Peters CA, eds. *Campbell-Walsh Urology*. 9th ed. Philadelphia, PA: Saunders Elsevier Company; 2007:788–801.

20. Lazarou S. Surgical treatment of erectile dysfunction. *UpToDate*. 2009.

21. Montague DK. Prosthetic surgery for erectile dysfunction In: Wein AJ, Kavoussi LR, Novick AC, Partin AW, Peters CA, eds. *Campbell-Walsh Urology*. 9th ed. Philadelphia, PA: Saunders Elsevier Company; 2007:788–801.

22. Montague DK. Prosthetic surgery for erectile dysfunction. In: Wein AJ, Kavoussi LR, Novick AC, Partin AW, Peters CA, eds. *Campbell-Walsh Urology*. 9th ed. Philadelphia, PA: Saunders Elsevier Company; 2007:788–801.

23. Jarow JP. Risk factors for penile prosthetic infection. *J Urol*. 1996;156:402.

24. Wilson SK, Carson CC, Cleves MA, Delk JR. Quantifying risks of penile prosthesis infection with elevated glycosylated hemoglobin. *J Urol*. 1998;159:1537.

25. Dos Reis JM, Glina S, Da Silva MF, Furlan V. Penile prosthesis surgery with the patient under local regional anesthesia. *J Urol*. 1993;150:1179.

26. D'Amico DF, Parimbelli P, Ruffolo C. Antibiotic prophylaxis in clean surgery: breast surgery and hernia repair. *J Chemother*. 2001;13(Spec 1):108.

27. Montague DK. Prosthetic surgery for erectile dysfunction. In: Wein AJ, Kavoussi LR, Novick AC, Partin AW, Peters CA, eds. *Campbell-Walsh Urology*. 9th ed. Philadelphia, PA: Saunders Elsevier Company; 2007:788–801.

28. Lazarou S. Surgical treatment of erectile dysfunction. *UpToDate*. 2009.

29. Montague DK. Prosthetic surgery for erectile dysfunction. In: Wein AJ, Kavoussi LR, Novick AC, Partin AW, Peters CA, eds. *Campbell-Walsh Urology*. 9th ed. Philadelphia, PA: Saunders Elsevier Company; 2007:788–801.

30. Lazarou S. Surgical treatment of erectile dysfunction. *UpToDate*. 2009.

31. Jarow JP. Risk factors for penile prosthetic infection. *J Urol*. 1996;156:402.

32. Wilson SK, Delk JR 2nd. Inflatable penile implant infection: predisposing factors and treatment suggestions. *J Urol*. 1995;153:659.

33. Montague DK: Prosthetic surgery for erectile dysfunction. In: Wein AJ, Kavoussi LR, Novick AC, Partin AW, Peters CA, eds. *Campbell–Walsh Urology*. 9th ed. Philadelphia, PA: Saunders Elsevier Company; 2007:788–801.

34. Abouassaly R, Montague DK, Angermeier KW. Antibiotic-coated medical devices: with an emphasis on inflatable penile prostheses. *Asian J Androl*. 2004;6:249–257.

35. Montague DK. Prosthetic surgery for erectile dysfunction. In: Wein AJ, Kavoussi LR, Novick AC, Partin AW, Peters CA, eds. *Campbell-Walsh Urology*. 9th ed. Philadelphia, PA: Saunders Elsevier Company; 2007:788–801.

36. Montague DK. Prosthetic surgery for erectile dysfunction. In: Wein AJ, Kavoussi LR, Novick AC, Partin AW, Peters CA, eds. *Campbell-Walsh Urology*. 9th ed. Philadelphia, PA: Saunders Elsevier Company; 2007:788–801.

37. Mulcahy JJ. Long-term experience with salvage of infected penile implants. *J Urol*. 2000;163:481–482.

38. Montague DK, Angermeier KW. Penile prosthesis implantation. *Urol Clin North America*. 2001;28:355.

39. Michal V, Kramar R, Pospichal J, Hejhal L. Direct arterial anastomosis to the cavernous body in the treatment of erectile impotence. *Rozhl Chir*. 1973;52:587–592.

40. Virag R, Bennett AH. Arterial and venous surgery for vasculogenic impotence: a combined French and American experience. *J Urol*. 1986;135:699–702.

41. Crespo EL, Soltanik E, Bove D, Farrell G. Treatment of vasculogenic sexual impotence by revascularization of cavernous and/or dorsal arteries using microvascular techniques. *Urology*. 1982;20:271–279.

42. Goldstein I. Overview of types and results of vascular surgical procedures for impotence. *Cardiovasc Interv Radiol.* 1988;11:240.
43. DePalma RG, Olding M, Yu GW, et al. Vascular interventions for impotence: lessons learned. *J Vasc Surg.* 1995;21: 576.
44. Vardi Y, Gruenwald I, Gedalia U, et al. Evaluation of penile revascularization for erectile dysfunction: a 10-year follow-up. *Int J Impot Res.* 2004;16:181.

CHAPTER 6

Peyronie's Disease

Adam Luchey, MD ■ *Stanley Zaslau, MD, MBA, FACS*

■ Introduction

- Named after François Gigot de la Peyronie in 1741, Peyronie's disease (PD), a benign condition, is characterized by a palpable plaque and curvature of the penis when erect.
- Lindsay et al. published the results of a 35-year study that showed a prevalence of 0.4% and the average age of onset at 53 years.[1]
- However, when studied in autopsies, Smith noted the prevalence of plaques to be 22 of 100 men.
- More recently, a review by Jalkut et al. stated that the increasing number of men presenting today with Peyronie's disease can be attributed to the role of phosphodiesterase inhibitors in treatment for erectile dysfunction. Thus, an underlying ED may be responsible for the development of Peyronie's disease.
- Although no specific cause can be attributed to Peyronie's disease, sexual trauma is strongly suspected.
  - Trauma to the tunica albuginea allows release of transforming growth factor, activating reactive oxygen species, which allows collagen deposits and calcification of the plaque that causes the deformity.[3]

■ Physical Examination

- Peyronie's disease is divided into two phases, the acute and the chronic phase.
- The acute phase is characterized by:
  - Painful erections
  - Nodule formation
  - Change in curvature of erection (up to the first 18 months)

- The chronic phase is characterized by:
  - Stable nodule and deformity
  - Relief of discomfort[4,5]
- Peyronie's disease can cause erectile dysfunction in up to 30–50% of cases and can prevent the patient from engaging in sexual intercourse.
- Photographs of the erections are helpful, especially for following changes with treatment and planning any operative management.
- The majority of the plaques are located on the dorsal or lateral sides of the penis.
- When talking with patients, the practitioner should inquire about other risk factors that may cause erectile dysfunction, such as:
  - Diabetes
  - Smoking
  - Hyperlipidemia
  - Hypertension
  - Coronary artery disease
- Some believe there is an association between Peyronie's disease and Dupuytren's contractures, which should also be evaluated on physical exam.
- Examining the penis in an outstretched position can help identify the extent of the plaques.
- Ultrasound can help identify any calcification and can aid in tracking progression and/or response to treatment.

■ Medical Therapy

Vitamin E

- Vitamin E is an antioxidant, which means it inhibits oxidation by free radicals (**Table 6.1**).
- However, it has a few side effects:
  - Treatment can increase the likelihood of heart failure
  - Has anticoagulative effects
- Recent studies fail to show significant clinical benefit.[8]
- This agent is given in divided doses of 800–1000 units per day. Typically Vitamin E is used for less than six months.

Table 6.1 Treatments for Peyronie's Disease

	Pros	Cons
Vitamin E	Antioxidant, scavenger of free radicals, few side effects	Recent studies fail to show benefit.[6,7] Treatment can potentiate heart failure and anticoagulative effects.
Aminobenzoate Potassium	Possibly decrease fibrinogenesis through altering serotonin levels[4]	Expensive, GI upset. Other studies have shown no benefit of correcting deformity; not recommended.[9,10,11]
Colchicine	Small, noncontrolled, unblinded shown benefit of improving curvature and decreasing plaque size[12]	Check periodic CBC (can lower blood cell counts), diarrhea
Tamoxifen	Regulated immune response through TGF-B decreasing fibrinogenesis[13]	Alopecia, no difference between tamoxifen and placebo[15]
Carnitine	Showed promise when compared to tamoxifen	Not recommended when compared to placebo[16]
Intralesional Verapamil	Decrease in plaque volume and possible decrease in curvature deformity through inhibiting exocytosis of collagen, fibronectin, and glycosaminoglycans (increase collagenase activity)[14]	Only benefits acute phase. Topical verapamil not recommended.[17]
ESWT	Hypothesize plaque lysis through inflammatory macrophages.	No improvement in curvature, plaque size, or sexual function.[18,19]

Dosage

- Vitamin E: Divided doses of 800–1000 units per day.
- Aminobenzoate Potassium: 12 g/day in 4–6 divided doses[6]
- Colchicine: 0.6 mg–1.2 mg daily for first week to 2.4 mg daily for three months in divided doses
- Tamoxifen: 20 mg twice daily
- Carnitine: 1 gram twice daily
- Intralesional Verapamil: 12 injections (10 mg/ml) per day for two to four weeks

Abern and Levine studied intralesional steroids, which showed no objective benefit, and collagenase, which showed a possible benefit in plaque width and curvature; further studies are ongoing. The same researchers also showed promising results from taking combination intralesional verapamil with traction and oral pentoxifylline and L-arginine.[11]

■ Surgical Therapy

- This procedure is not appropriate during the acute phase (< 1 years, painful erections) when the plaque is still changing and not mature. Three procedures are considered to be commonly performed depending on the degree and location of the plaque. These are:
  1. Nesbitt procedure
  2. Plaque excision and graft interposition
  3. Penile prosthesis placement and orthoplasty

Nesbit Procedure

Nesbit procedure was first described in 1965 for correction of congenital curvature.[20] When performing the Nesbit procedure, an elliptical incision is made into the tunica albuginea opposite that from the plaque in order to straighten the curvature.

- Patients are told pre-operatively that they will experience penile shortening on average of 0.5 cm but values greater than this have been reported. In addition, details on loss of sensation, hematoma, and urethral injury have to be included.

- Akkus et al., which published recommendations from 10 experts, stated that the Nesbit procedure was the treatment of choice with the least risk of postoperative erectile dysfunction for a stable deformity.[21]

- Through modification of the procedure, Rolle et al. were able to achieve a statistical improvement in erectile dysfunction through a modified corporoplasty that enabled them to excise the fibrosed tunica albuginea only after the correct position was determined in real time without lengthening the operation. This was proven in both acquired and congenital penile curvature.[22]

Plaque Excision and Graft Interposition

- In general, graft material (buccal, saphenous vein, tunica vaginalis, fascia lata, rectus fascia, cadaveric, and bovine pericardium) has less of a risk of penile shortening than other surgical procedure but the risk of erectile dysfunction is greater.

- Buccal mucosa has been shown to have no shrinkage or change in elasticity and Liu et al. achieved complete straightening in 21 of 24 patients followed for 0.5–7 years with minimal loss of length.[23]

- In a retrospective analysis of 11 patients undergoing dermal grafting, were encouraged to achieve erections after two weeks and sexual intercourse after six weeks.[24]

- In a head to head comparison between cadaveric pericardium and dermal grafts, Chun and McGregor et al. showed that cadaveric pericardial grafts are equal to dermal grafts with the added benefit of commercial availability without the need for harvesting.[25]

Penile Prosthesis Placement with Orthoplasty

Prosthesis involvement for Peyronie's is best suited for the elderly male with significant curvature as well as severe erectile dysfunction, and for this it is considered the first-line of treatment.[26]

- Older prostheses did not allow modeling because their length did not achieve the rigidity needed to correct curvature. With advances in penile prostheses their applicability in Peyronie's grew.

Ghanem et al. studied 20 men who had malleable penile prosthesis placed, all of which failed intracavernous injections. They reported straightening of the penile shaft in all cases and all but two were satisfied at one year post-op.[27]

- Carson and colleagues studies 30 men, all with their duration of deformity greater than 12 months who were able to achieve penile straightening with a functional implant and modeling in 28 patients; the remaining required plaque incision.[28] It has been known that modeling over an implant lends to an increase in intra-operative urethral injury compared to implantation of prosthesis by itself.[29]

- There is no one perfect operation for chronic Peyronie's disease. The physician must take into account the underlying erectile function, or lack thereof, and the risk of penile shortening when determining their approach. As always, surgeon experience is critical to patient outcome.

■ Conclusions

- Although no specific cause of Peyronie's disease is fully known, sexual trauma is strongly suspected.

- Peyronie's disease can cause ED and can prevent the patient from engaging in sexual intercourse.

- Medical and surgical therapies are available to treat Peryonie's disease. Treatment must be individualized to the patient's degree of curvature, location of curvature, and presence of underlying ED.

- Treatment is currently evolving and continued research in this area is ongoing.

■ References

1. Lindsay MB, Schain DM, Grambasch P. The incidence of Peyronie's disease in Rochester, Minnesota, 1950 through 1984. *J Urol*. 1991;146:1007–1009.

2. Smith BH. Subclinical Peyronie's disease. *Am J Clin Pathol*. 1969;52:385–390.

3. Jalkut M, Gonzalez-Cadavid N, Rajfer J. Peyronie's disease: a review. *Rev Urol*. 2003 Summer;5(3):142–148.

4. Hellstrom WJ. Medical management of Peyronie's disease. *J Androl.* 2009;30:397–405.

5. Gelbard MK, Dorey F, James K. The natural history of Peyronie's disease. *J Urol.* 1990;149:53–55.

6. Hasche-Klunder R. Treatment of Peyronie's disease with para-aminobenzoacidic potassium (POTABA). *Urologe A.* 1978;17:224–227.

7. Pryor JP, Farrell CF. Controlled clinical trial of vitamin E in Peyronie's disease. *Prog Reprod Biol.* 1983;9:41–45.

8. Broderick GA, Lue TF. Evaluation and nonsurgical management of erectile dysfunction and premature ejaculation. In: Wein AJ, Kavoussi LR, Novick AC, Partin AW, Peters CA, eds. *Campbell-Walsh Urology.* 9th ed. Philadelphia, PA: Saunders Elsevier Company; 2007:818–838.

9. Hasche-Klunder R. Treatment of Peyronie's disease with para-aminobenzoacidic potassium (POTABA). *Urologe A.* 1978 Jul;17(4):224–227.

10. Weidner W, Hauch EW, Schnitker J. Peyronie's disease study group of andrological group of german urologists. Potassium paraaminobenzoate (Potaba) in the treatment of Peyronie's disease: a prospective, placebo-controlled, randomized study. *Eur Urol.* 2005;47:530–536.

11. Abern M, Levine L. Peyronie's disease: evaluation and review of nonsurgical therapy. *TSWJ.* 2009 Jul 27;9:665–675.

12. Akkus E, Carrier S, Rehman J, et al. Is colchicine effective in Peyronie's disease? A pilot study. *Urology.* 1994;44:291–295.

13. Colletta A, Wakefield L, Howell F, et al. Anti-oestrogens induce the secretion of transforming growth factor beta from human fetal fibroblasts. *Br J Cancer.* 1990;62:405–409.

14. Levine LA, Goldman K, Greenfield J. Experience with intraplaque injections of verapamil injection. *J Urol.* 1997;158:1395–1399.

15. Telojen C, Rhoden E, Grazziotin T, et al. Tamoxifen versus placebo in the treatment of Peyronie's disease. *J Urol.* 1999;162:2003–2005.

16. Safarinejad M, Hosseini S, Kolahi A. Comparison of vitamin E and propionyl-L-carnitine, separately or in combination, in patients with early chronic Peyronie's disease: a double-blind, placebo controlled, randomized study. *J Urol.* 2007;178:1398–1403.

17. Levine L. Comment on topical verapamil HCl, topical trifluoperazine, and topical magnesium sulfate for the treat-

ment of Peyronie's disease—a placebo-controlled pilot study. *J Sex Med.* 2007;4:1081–1082.

18. Hatzichristodoulou G, Mesiner C, Stenzl A, et al. (2006) *Efficacy of extracorporeal shock wave therapy (ESWT) in patients with Peyronie's disease (PD)—first results of a prospective, randomized, placebo-controlled study.* Paper presented at the AUA meeting.

19. Hatzichristodoulou G, Mesiner C, Stenzl A, et al. (2006) Efficacy of extracorporeal shock wave therapy (ESWT) in patients with Peyronie's disease (PD)—first results of a prospective, randomized, placebo-controlled study. Paper presented at the AUA meeting.

20. Nesbit RM. Congenital curvature of the phallus report of three cases with description of corrective operation. *J Urol.* 1965;93:230.

21. Pryor J, Akkus E, Alter G, Jordan G, Lebret T, Levine L, et al. Peyronie's disease. *J Sex Med.* 2004;1:110–115.

22. Rolle L, Tamagnone AT, Timpano M, et al. The Nesbit operation for penile curvature: an easy and effective technical modification. *J Urol.* 2005;173:171–174.

23. Liu B, Zhu XW, Zhong DC, Shen BH, Jiang H, Xie LP. Replacement of plaque by buccal mucosa in the treatment of Peyronie's disease: a report of 27 cases. *Zhonghua Nan Ke Xue.* 2009;15:45–47.

24. Royal NK, Kumar A, Das SK, Pandey AK, Sharma GK, Trivedi S, Dwivedi US. Experience with plaque excision and dermal grafting in the surgical treatment of Peyronie's disease. *Singapore Med J.* 2008;48:805–808.

25. Chun J, McGregor A, Krishnan R, Carson C. A comparison of dermal and cadaveric pericardial grafts in the modified Horton-Devine procedure for Peyronie's disease. *J Urol.* 2001;166:185–188.

26. Levine LA, Lenting EL. A surgical algorithm for the treatment of Peyronie's disease. *J Urol.* 1997;158:2149–2152.

27. Ghanem HM, Fahmy I, El-Meliegy A. Malleable penile implant without plauq surgery in the treatment of Peynoie's disease. *Int J Impotence Research.* 1998;10:171–174.

28. Carson CC. Penile prosthesis implantation in the treatment of Peyronie's Disease. *Int J Impotence Research.* 1998;10:125–1258.

29. Wilson S, Cleves M, Delk J. Long-term followup of treatment for Peyronie's Disease: modeling the penis over an inflatable penile prosthesis. *J Urol.* 2001;165:825–829.

SECTION 2

Female Sexual Dysfunction

Physiology of Female Sexual Function

Chad P. Hubsher, MD ■ *Adam Luchey, MD* ■ *Stanley Zaslau, MD, MBA, FACS*

■ Introduction

- Sexual function in women is a highly variable, multi-faceted process involving several components:
  - Anatomical
  - Physiological
  - Psychological
  - Emotional
  - Interpersonal
- Given the complex nature of sexuality in females, little consensus currently exists on the definition of a "normal sexual response."
- Although aspects of female sexual function, such as vaginal lubrication and orgasmic contractions, seem to be widespread in normal, sexually functioning women, the subjective or emotional aspects are highly individual. These aspects are subject to learning and cultural factors, as past experiences play an important role in shaping expectations regarding sexual response in women.

■ Female Sexual Response Cycle

- Over the past 45 years, several models have been proposed to aid in the understanding of the female sexual response cycle.
- These models provide a conceptual framework of the sequence of physiological events and psychological processes that comprise normal sexual response for most

women. However, to date, none of the proposed female sexual response models have been shown to be universally applicable.

The Masters and Johnson (Four-Stage) Model

- Masters and Johnson first characterized the female sexual response cycle in 1966 based on laboratory observations of approximately 700 men and women.[1]
- They proposed a model of female sexual response consisting of four successive phases, each of which has associated genital and extragenital responses (**Figure 7.1**):
  - Excitement
  - Plateau
  - Orgasm
  - Resolution

The Three-Stage Model

- In 1974, Kaplan proposed a three-stage model that acknowledged the importance of subjective, psychological, and interpersonal aspects of sexual response.[2]
- In this model, the sexual response cycle was reconceptualized to consist of three essential phases:
  - Desire
  - Arousal
  - Orgasm
- This three-stage model was used in the fourth edition of the *Diagnostic and Statistical Manual of Mental Disorders* (DSM-IV) as the basis for the classification of female sexual dysfunction. It was also used in the American Foundation of Urologic Disease's 1998 reclassification per their first international consensus development panel on female sexual dysfunction.[3]

■ Female Sexual Anatomy

- In order to adequately understand female sexual function, it is necessary to have a formal understanding of the female pelvic anatomy.

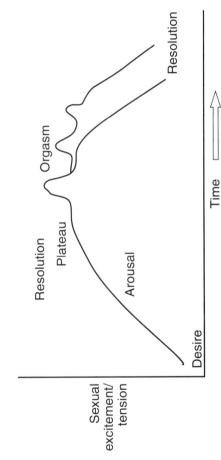

Figure 7.1 The Masters and Johnson Model
Source: Adapted from Masters WH & Johnson VE. *Human Sexual Response.* Boston, MA: Little Brown & Co,; 1966.

- The organs and structures can be grouped into external and internal genitalia.
  - The external genitalia, collectively known as the vulva, consist of:
    - The labial formation
    - Interlabial space
    - Erectile tissues, including the clitoris and vestibular bulbs
  - They are bound anteriorly by the pubic symphysis, laterally by the ischial tuberosities, and posteriorly by the anal sphincter.
  - The internal genitalia consist of the:
    - Vagina
    - Uterus
    - Fallopian tubes
    - Ovaries
    - Pelvic floor muscles

Labial Formation

- The labial formation is designed to provide protection to the urethral and vaginal orifices, both of which open into the vestibule of the vagina.
- It consists of two pairs of symmetrically folded skin; the outer folds, known as the labia majora, fuse with each other anteriorly at the anterior labial commissure, while the inner folds, known as the labia minora, are continuous with the vaginal mucosa and fuse together to form the prepuce of the clitoris anteriorly, and the frenulum posteriorly.
- The labia majora are composed of subcutaneous fat and covered by hair-bearing skin, while the labia minora are covered by hairless skin and are composed of a fat-free spongy tissue punctuated by sebaceous and sweat glands along with many blood vessels and sensory nerve endings.
- The labial formation is innervated by the perineal and posterior labial branches of the pudendal nerve. The arterial blood supply is derived from the inferior perineal and posterior labial branches of the pudendal artery, as well as superficial branches of the femoral artery.

Interlabial Space

- The area medial to the labia minora, bound anteriorly by the clitoris and posteriorly by the frenulum, is known as the interlabial space.
- The urethral orifice, vaginal orifice, and greater vestibular gland, also known as Bartholin glands, all open into this space.
  - The greater vestibular glands are located in the superficial perineal pouch, underneath the bulbs of the vestibule, and secrete a small amount of lubricating mucus into the vestibule of the vagina during sexual arousal.

Clitoris

- The clitoris is an erectile organ similar to the penis that arises from the same embryological structure, the genital tubercle.
- It is cylindrical in shape, located posterior to the anterior labial commissure, and composed of three parts:
  - The outermost glans or head
  - The middle corpus or body
  - The innermost crura
- The glans clitoris is often hidden by the labial formations when nonengorged, but may be visualized as it emerges from the labia minora.
- The body of the clitoris extends beneath the skin and gives rise to bilateral crura, called corpora cavernosa, which, similar to the penis, are composed of erectile tissue and separated by a septum.
- The paired crura of the clitoris are homologous to the male corpora and are comprised of:
  - Lacunar sinusoids
  - A trabecula of vascular smooth muscle
  - A collagen connective tissue surrounded by a thick fibrous sheath known as the tunica albuginea
- Unlike the bilaminar structure found in the penis, the tunica albuginea in the clitoris is unilaminar. There is thus no mechanism for venous trapping in the clitoris and as a result, sexual stimulation produces clitoral engorgement, not erection, as is seen in the penis.

- During sexual stimulation, blood flow to the clitoris almost doubles, resulting in an increase in length and diameter, as was demonstrated by Park and colleagues using duplex ultrasounds.[4]
- The iliohypogastric arterial bed is the main arterial supply to the clitoris. The internal iliac artery traverses the pudendal canal (Alcock's canal), after it gives off its last anterior branch, the internal pudendal artery.
  - The internal iliac then terminates as the common clitoral artery, which gives off the dorsal clitoral artery and clitoral cavernosal arteries.
  - It is these arteries that are responsible for engorgement of the corporeal bodies upon sexual stimulation and arousal.
- The nerve endings located in the clitoris are comprised of autonomic and somatic innervation.
  - The autonomic innervation of the clitoris is formed by the pelvic and hypogastric plexuses. These plexuses carry sympathetic (T1-L3) and parasympathetic (S2-S4) fibers that join together at the base of the broad ligament, on each side of the supravaginal part of the cervix, to form the uterovaginal plexus and send direct fibers to both the clitoris and vagina.
  - Somatic sensory innervation of the clitoris arises in the skin and travels to the sacral spinal cord via the dorsal nerve of the clitoris and pudendal nerve.
- Within the clitoris there is a dense collection of Pacinian corpuscles, Meissner's corpuscles, and Merkel tactile disks, which are responsible for transmitting information to the brain concerning pain and pressure, light touch, and texture, respectively.

Vestibular Bulbs

- The other erectile tissues of the female genitalia are the vestibular bulbs.
- These are 3-cm-long paired structures that lie beneath the skin of the labia minora, directly along the sides of the vaginal orifices.
- They are homologous to the corpus spongiosum of the penis. However, unlike the penis, the vestibular bulbs

are separated from the clitoris, urethra, and vestibule of the vagina.

- The recent cadaver dissections of O'Connell and associates revealed that the bulbs lie on the superficial aspect of the vaginal wall, not forming the core of the labia minora. They also discovered that there are considerable age-related variations in the dimensions of the vestibular bulbs in young, premenopausal women versus older, postmenopausal women.[5]

Vagina

- The vagina is a midline cylindrical organ that is approximately 7–9 cm in length.
- It extends from the cervix of the uterus to the vestibule of the vagina, and its walls are composed of four layers:
  - An inner mucosal layer
    - The inner vaginal mucosa is a stratified squamous nonkeratinized mucus type epithelium that undergoes hormone-related cyclical changes during the menstrual cycle in which a slight keratinization of the superficial cells occurs.
  - A lamina propia
    - The lamina propia separates the mucosal layer and the muscularis.
  - A muscularis layer
    - The vaginal muscularis is composed of outer longitudinal and inner smooth muscle cell fibers, as well as an extensive tree of blood vessels.
  - An outer adventitial supportive mesh layer
    - The surrounding outermost fibrous layer is rich in collagen, and provides structural support to the vagina. It is this outermost layer that is responsible for expansion of the vagina during childbirth and intercourse.
- During sexual arousal, there is increased blood flow to the subepithelial blood vessels, resulting in genital vasocongestion and subsequent engorgement of the vaginal wall.
- According to Levin, the increase in pressure inside the subepithelial vascular bed results in passive transudation of plasma through the vaginal epithelium.[6] Along with

secretions from the uterine glands, this helps lubricate the vaginal canal.

- Initially, as the vaginal lubricative plasma flows onto the surface of the vagina, sweatlike droplets form. These eventually coalesce to create a lubricative film covering the vaginal wall.
- Further moistening during sexual arousal originates from secretions of the greater vestibular glands located in the interlabial space.

■ The nerve endings located in the vagina are comprised of autonomic and somatic innervation.

- The uterovaginal nerves, which originate from the hypogastric and sacral plexuses, contain both parasympathetic and sympathetic fibers, and supply autonomic innervation to the proximal two-thirds of the vagina, as well as the corporeal bodies of the clitoris.
- The uterovaginal nerve fibers, which travel within the uterosacral and cardinal ligaments before reaching the vagina, play a major role in sexual function, and thus serve as a potential site of injury and resultant sexual dysfunction from female pelvic surgery.
- The somatic sensory innervation of the vagina is primarily provided by the pudendal nerve.

■ The arterial supply to the vagina varies by location. Vaginal branches of the uterine artery supply the superior aspect of the vagina, the hypogastric artery supplies the middle vagina, and branches of the middle hemorrhoidal and clitoral arteries supply the distal aspect of the vagina.

Uterus

■ The uterus is a midline, mobile organ located between the rectum and urinary bladder that connects with the proximal aspect of the vaginal canal via the cervical os.

■ During sexual arousal, uterine and cervical glands secrete mucus to help lubricate the vaginal canal.

■ Surgical menopause, brought on by hysterectomy with oophorectomy, significantly impacts sexual function.

- Furthermore, as described by Carlson, hysterectomy alone, without removal of the ovaries, can also result in sexual dysfunction postoperatively.[7] Removal of the uterus disrupts the pelvic autonomic and cervical plexus, as well as the uterosacral and cardinal ligaments and the associated autonomic fibers. As previously discussed, this disturbs innervation to the vagina and clitoris, resulting in alteration in sexual function.

Pelvic Floor Muscles

- The pelvic floor is a collection of tissues that span the opening within the bony pelvis and function to:
  - Support the abdominal and pelvic organs
  - Maintain continence of urine and stool
  - Allow for parturition and intercourse
- Pelvic support is primarily provided by the levator ani muscles, urogenital diaphragm, and the perineal membrane, which consists of the ischiocavernosus, bulbocavernosus, and superficial transverse perineal muscles.
  - Voluntary contraction of the perineal membrane plays a role in sexual response by intensifying orgasm of both the female and male partner.
- The pelvic floor muscles can also cause sexual dysfunction.
  - At times, nonvoluntary pelvic floor spasms are associated with vaginal penetration.
  - Laxity and hypotonia of the pelvic floor result in symptoms of vaginal anesthesia, coital anorgasmia, and incontinence during intercourse or orgasm.
  - Women with pelvic floor disorders often present with coexisting urological and sexual complaints.

■ Female Sexual Response

- The female sexual response cycle, described earlier, is initiated by neurotransmitter-mediated vascular and nonvascular smooth muscle relaxation. The result is:
  - Increased pelvic blood flow
  - Vaginal lubrication
  - Clitoral and labial engorgement
- These mechanisms are mediated by a combination of neuromuscular and vasocongestive events that are under neurogenic and hormonal regulation.

■ Physiology of Sexual Arousal

- Sexual arousal in the female is associated with a variety of changes in the female sexual anatomy.
- The increase in pelvic blood flow via the iliohypogastric arterial bed, and simultaneous relaxation of the vaginal wall and clitoral cavernosal smooth muscle, is responsible for the observed engorgement of the labia minora, vagina, and clitoris during sexual arousal.
  - In the labia minora, the increase in blood flow, especially to the vestibular bulbs that lie directly beneath the skin of the labia, result in a two- to threefold increase in diameter of the labia, along with eversion and exposure of its inner surface.
  - In the vagina, the infiltration of blood in the extensive vasculature of the muscularis layer leads to vaginal wall engorgement and a concomitant expansion of the outermost fibrous layer to allow continued structural support of the vaginal canal.
  - Via the clitoral cavernosal arteries, the clitoris also experiences an enhancement blood flow during sexual arousal. The resultant increase in intracavernous pressure leads to extrusion and tumescence of the glans clitoris, unlike the rigidity as seen in the male penis.
    - Goldstein and Berman reported that unlike the penis, the clitoris lacks a subalbugineal layer between the tunica albuginea and erectile tissue.[8]
    - The subalbugineal layer in the male contains a rich venous plexus, and with sexual arousal, will expand against the tunica albuginea, causing a reduction in venous outflow and inducing rigidity in the penis.
    - Consequently, the absence of this venous plexus and subalbugineal layer in the clitoris allows only tumescence to be obtained.
- Increased lubrication of the vaginal canal during sexual arousal is achieved primarily via two mechanisms: transudate originating from the subepithelial vascular bed and secretions from uterine glands.
  - As previously described, vaginal engorgement enables a process of plasma transudation to occur, in which

increased pressure within the blood vessel helps transudate to form and plasma to flow through the epithelium and eventually create a lubricative film that covers the vaginal wall.

- Additional vaginal canal moistening during sexual arousal comes from secretions of the greater vestibular glands (Bartholin's glands).
- Furthermore, as reported by Toesca and colleagues, these secretions may also serve as a mechanism to attract the male sex by emitting fluid that is odiferous.[9]

Neurogenic Mediators

- Which and how neurotransmitters modulate vaginal and clitoral smooth muscle tone are currently being investigated.
- Recently, Burnett and colleagues and Hilliges and colleagues identified nitrous oxide (NO) and phosphodiesterase type 5 (PDE-5) in both clitoral and cavernosal smooth muscle.[10,11]
  - PDE-5 is the enzyme responsible for the degradation of cGMP, as well as formation of NO.
  - These neurotransmitters may serve as a potential therapeutic site for sexual dysfunction.
    - Vemulapalli and Kurowski determined that sildenafil, a specific PDE-5 inhibitor, causes dose-dependent relaxation of female rabbit clitoral and vaginal smooth muscle in organ bath studies.[12]
- Park and associates suggest that NO, in combination with vasoactive intestinal peptide (VIP), are involved in regulation of vaginal secretory processes and relaxation.[13]
  - VIP is a nonadrenergic, noncholinergic neurotransmitter that has been described by Levin to enhance vaginal blood flow, lubrication, and secretions.[14]
  - Similar to the aforementioned studies performed with PDE-5, Ziessen and colleagues determined that VIP causes dose-dependent relaxation of rabbit clitoral cavernosum and vaginal smooth muscle in organ bath studies.[15]
    - Thus, in addition to NO and PDE-5, there may be a role of endogenous VIP as a neurotransmitter in

clitoral and vaginal tissue and a mediator of female sexual response.

Hormonal Regulators

- Female sexual function is greatly affected by the levels of hormones in the body, specifically estrogen and testosterone.

Estrogen

- As was demonstrated by Natoin and associates, estrogens have vasoprotective and vasodilatory effects that increase arterial blood flow to the vagina, clitoris, and urethra.[16]
  - This prevents atherosclerotic compromise to the ilio-hypogastric arterial bed and thus helps maintain the female sexual response.
- Sarrel found that a decline in circulating estrogen levels, either due to aging or surgical castration, results in increased vaginal wall fibrosis caused by decreased vaginal NO levels.[17] This is because estrogen regulates nitric oxide synthase (NOS), the enzyme responsible for production of NO.
- Furthermore, it has been demonstrated that estrogen replacement therapy:
  - Increases vaginal NOS expression and NO levels
  - Restores vaginal mucosa
  - Decreases vaginal mucosal cell death
- In addition to having a significant role in preserving vaginal mucosa, estrogen is important in the maintenance and function of the vaginal epithelium and smooth muscle cells of the muscularis, and in lubrication of the vaginal canal.
- In fact, in animal studies performed by Berman and colleagues, a decline in the level of estrogen results in a less acidic vaginal environment and thinner and drier vaginal walls that damage more easily.[18]
  - These results likely correlate with complaints of female sexual dysfunction, including vaginal dryness and dyspareunia, often seen in women with a decline in circulating estrogen levels observed during aging and menopause.

Testosterone

- Similar to estrogen, testosterone also has a significant effect on female sexual function; however, the role of androgens remains controversial, as little is understood about their exact mechanism.
- Nonetheless, low levels of testosterone are associated with a decrease in:
  - Libido
  - Sexual arousal
  - Sexual responsiveness
  - Genital sensation
  - Orgasm
- In a study by Sherwin and Gelfand, menopausal women responded better to estrogen-androgen combinations compared to estrogen alone on measures of enhanced sexual desire, sexual arousal, enjoyment of sex, and number of orgasms.[19]
- In a study by Shifren and associates of women with hypothalamic amenorrhea, testosterone increased vaginal vasocongestion, as measured by plethysmography during exposure to a potent visual stimulus.[20]
- While pharmacological doses of testosterone have been shown to improve overall female sexual function, it is not known whether physiological testosterone replacement will produce clinically meaningful changes.
- Additionally, all androgens carry the risk of inducing virilization in women. Early reversible manifestations include acne, hirsutism, and menstrual irregularities, while long-term side effects are often irreversible, including male-pattern baldness, hypertrophy of the clitoris, and voice changes.

■ Conclusions

- Although there are significant anatomical, embryological, and physiological parallels between men and women, it is important to have a clear understanding of the differences.
- The multifaceted nature of female sexuality further contributes to the complexity in differentiating a normal sexual response from female sexual dysfunction.

■ References

1. Masters WH, Johnson VE. *Human Sexual Response*. Boston, MA: Little, Brown & Co.; 1966.

2. Kaplan HS. *The New Sex Therapy*. London, England: Bailliere Tindall; 1974.

3. Basson R, Berman J, Burnett A, et al. Report of the international consensus development conference on female sexual dysfunction: definitions and classifications. *J Urol.* 2000;163:888–893.

4. Park K, Goldstein I, Andry C, Siroky MB, Krane RJ, Azadzoi KM. Vasculogenic female sexual dysfunction: the hemodynamic basis for vaginal engorgement insufficiency and clitoral erectile insufficiency. *Int J Impot Res.* 1997;9:27–37.

5. O'Connell HE, Hutson JM, Anderson CR, Plenter RJ. Anatomical relationship between urethra and clitoris. *J Urol.* 1998;159:1892–1897.

6. Levin RJ. The physiology of sexual function in women. *Clin Obstet Gynecol.* 1980;7:213–252.

7. Carlson KJ. Outcomes of hysterectomy. *Clin Obstet Gynecol.* 1997;40:939–940.

8. Goldstein I, Berman JR: Vasculogenic female sexual dysfunction: vaginal engorgement and clitoral erectile insufficiency syndromes. *Int J Impot Rs.* 1998;10:S84–S90.

9. Toesca A, Stolfi VM, Cocchia D. Immunohistochemical study of the corpora cavernosa of the human clitoris. *J Anat.* 1996;188:513–520.

10. Burnett AL, Calvin DC, Silver RI, Peppas DS, Docimo SG. Immunohistochemical description of nitric oxide synthase isoforms in human clitoris. *J Urol.* 1997;158:75–80.

11. Hilliges M, Falconer C, Ekman-Ordeberg G, Johanson O. Innervation of human vaginal mucosa as revealed by PGP 9.5 immunohistochemistry. *Acta Anat.* 1995;153:119–126.

12. Vemulapalli S, Kurowski S. Sildenafil relaxes rabbit clitoral corpus cavernosum. *Life Sci.* 2000;67:23–29.

13. Park K, Moreland RB, Goldstein I, Atala A, Traish A. Characterization of phosphodiesterase activity in human clitoral corpus cavernosum smooth muscle cells in culture. *Biochem Biophys Res Commun.* 1998;249:612–617.

14. Levin RJ. VIP, vagina, clitoral and periurethral glans: an update on female genital arousal. *Exp Clin Endocrinol.* 1991;98:61–69.

15. Ziessen T, Moncada S, Cellek S. Characterization of the non-nitrergic NANC relaxation responses in the rabbit vaginal wall. *Br J Pharmacol.* 2002;135:546–554.

16. Naftolin F, Maclusky NJ, Leranth CZ. The cellular effects of estrogens on neuroendocrine tissues. *J Steroid Biochem.* 1988;30:195–207.

17. Sarrel PM. Ovarian hormones and vaginal blood flow using laser Doppler velocimetry to measure effects in a clinical trial of postmenopausal women. *Int J Impot Res.* 1998;10:S91–S93.

18. Berman J, McCarthy M, Kyprianou N. Effect of estrogen withdrawal in nitric oxide synthase expression and apoptosis in the rat vagina. *Urology.* 1998;44:650–656.

19. Sherwin BB, Gelfand MM. Differential symptom response to parental estrogen and androgen in the surgical menopause. *Am J Obstet Gynecol.* 1985;151:153–160.

20. Shifren JL, Braunstein GD, Simon JA, et al. Transdermal testosterone treatment in women with impaired sexual function after oophorectomy. *N Engl J Med.* 2000;343:682–688.

CHAPTER 8

Classification and Pathogenesis of Female Sexual Dysfunction

Chad P. Hubsher, MD ■ *Aimee Rogers, MD* ■ *Stanley Zaslau, MD, MBA, FACS*

■ Introduction and Classification

- Sexual dysfunction in the female population is a highly prevalent, multidimensional problem that combines biological, psychological, and interpersonal determinants.

- Approximately 40% of women experience sexual complaints. The Global Study of Sexual Attitudes and Behaviors identified that 26–43% and 18–41% of females 40–80 years old worldwide experience a low sexual desire and inability to reach orgasm, respectively.

- Laumann and colleagues conducted an analysis of the National Health and Social Life Survey, a probability sample study of sexual behavior in a demographically representative cohort of the United States.[1] They found that:

  - Between the ages of 18 and 59, sexual dysfunction is more prevalent in women (43%) than men (31%), and married women are less likely to experience decreased sexual desire and pleasure than unmarried women.

  - African American women consistently reported the highest rates of sexual problems, whereas Hispanic women have lower rates of sexual dysfunction than do white women.

  - Sexual pain, however, is most likely to occur in white women.[1,2]

- Although this survey has limitations, including its age restriction, cross-sectional design, and failure to adjust for the effects of menopausal status or medical risk factors, it clearly indicates that sexual dysfunction affects many women.

- In contrast to male sexual dysfunction, female sexual dysfunction has only recently become widely recognized by the urological community.
- In 1998 the Sexual Function Health Council of the American Foundation of Urologic Disease organized the first international consensus development conference on female sexual dysfunction to evaluate, revise, and identify new definitions and classifications.[3]
  - Medical risk factors, etiologies, and psychological aspects were classified into four categories of female sexual dysfunction. Each of the diagnoses described below can be further subtyped as:
    - Lifelong versus acquired
    - Generalized versus situational
    - Etiologic origin of organic, psychogenic, mixed, or unknown
  - **Table 8.1** displays the classification of female sexual dysfunction. The following bullet points provide more detail on each of the disorders.

Sexual Desire Disorders

- There are two types of sexual desire disorders that contribute to female sexual dysfunction.
  - Hypoactive sexual desire disorder is the persistent or recurrent deficiency (or absence) of sexual

Table 8.1   Classification of Female Sexual Dysfunction

I. Sexual desire disorders:
   a. Hypoactive sexual desire disorder
   b. Sexual aversion disorder

II. Sexual arousal disorder

III. Orgasmic disorder

IV. Sexual pain disorders:
   a. Dyspareunia
   b. Vaginismus
   c. Other sexual pain disorders

fantasies/thoughts, and/or desire for or receptivity to sexual activity, which causes personal distress.

- It may result from emotional or psychological factors, such as lifestyle issues, including finances, careers, and family commitments, or it may be secondary to physiological problems, such as those caused by medical or surgical interventions and hormonal deficiencies. In fact, any disruption of the female hormonal environment, such as those caused by natural menopause, surgically or medically induced menopause, or endocrine disorders, may result in an inhibited sexual desire.

- Sexual aversion disorder is the persistent or recurrent inability to have, phobic aversion to, and avoidance of sexual contact with a sexual partner, which causes personal distress.

  - Unlike hypoactive sexual desire disorder, it is less likely to be related to physiological issues. Instead, it is often an emotional or psychologically based problem that can result from a variety of factors, including physical or sexual abuse or childhood trauma.

Sexual Arousal Disorder

- Sexual arousal disorder is the persistent or recurrent inability to attain or maintain sufficient sexual excitement, causing personal distress.
- It may be expressed as a lack of subjective excitement, or a lack of genital (lubrication/swelling) or other somatic responses.
- Disorders of arousal include, but are not limited to:
  - Decreased clitoral and labial engorgement
  - Diminished or lack of vaginal lubrication
  - Lack of relaxation of the vaginal smooth muscle
- These conditions may be caused by psychological factors, but more commonly have medical or physiological bases. Such etiologies include:
  - Prior pelvic trauma or surgery that may have disrupted the neurovasculature

- Decreased blood flow to the vagina and clitoris
- Medications, especially selective serotonin reuptake inhibitors

Orgasmic Disorder

- Orgasmic disorder is the persistent or recurrent difficulty of, delay in, or absence of attaining orgasm following sufficient sexual stimulation and arousal, which causes personal distress.
- This may be a primary condition, in which the woman has never achieved orgasm, or a secondary condition as a result of hormonal deficiencies, trauma, or surgery.
- Primary anorgasmia can be due to medical and physiological factors as well as sexual abuse or emotional trauma.

Sexual Pain Disorders

- In females, there are three classifications of pain disorders that contribute to sexual dysfunction.
  - Dyspareunia is recurrent or persistent genital pain associated with sexual intercourse. It can be due to physiological and/or psychological factors.
  - Pain with sexual intercourse can also develop secondary to irritative conditions such as friction as a result of inadequate lubrication, or medical problems, including vaginal infection, vaginal atrophy, or vestibulitis.
  - Vaginismus is the recurrent or persistent involuntary spasm of the musculature of the outer third of the vagina that interferes with vaginal penetration, and causes personal distress.
    - Vaginismus generally develops as a conditioned response to painful penetration.
    - It can also develop secondary to emotional or psychological factors.
    - Recurrent or persistent genital pain induced by noncoital sexual stimulation is referred to as noncoital sexual pain disorder.

■ Etiologies of Female Sexual Dysfunction

- The etiology of sexual dysfunction in women is often multifactorial, and may include:
  - Emotional issues relating to prior physical or sexual abuse or conflicts within the relationship
  - Psychological problems such as fatigue, stress, depression, or anxiety disorders
  - Physical problems that may make sexual activity uncomfortable
- Additionally, some medications and various medical conditions may significantly impair sexual function.
- The following sections describe each of these etiologies in more detail.

Vasculogenic

- In men, high blood pressure, heart disease, high cholesterol levels, diabetes, and smoking are associated with vasculogenic impotence. Similar to Leriche's syndrome in men, secondary to aortoiliac occlusive disease, clitoral and vaginal vascular insufficiency syndrome results from decreased inflow to the clitoris or vagina and is primarily due to atherosclerosis of the iliohypogastric and pudendal arterial bed.
- Park et al. further characterized this phenomenon and determined that the diminished pelvic blood flow leads to loss of corporal smooth muscle in the clitoris, with replacement by fibrous connective tissue, and atherosclerosis of clitoral cavernosal arteries.[4]
- In addition, any traumatic injury to the iliohypogastric pudendal arterial bed from surgical disruption, blunt trauma, pelvic fractures, or chronic perineal pressure, as may be seen from riding a bicycle for an extended period of time, can result in diminished vaginal and clitoral blood flow and result in sexual complaints.

Neurogenic

- The same neurological disorders that cause erectile dysfunction in men can also cause sexual dysfunction in women.

- Neurogenic female sexual dysfunction can result from spinal cord injury or disease of the central or peripheral nervous system, including diabetes and multiple sclerosis.
  - In fact, Hutler and Lundberg determined that 62% of women with advanced multiple sclerosis have sensory dysfunction in the genital region.[5]
  - Spinal cord injury does not always limit a woman's ability to become pregnant, but it may compromise female sexual function in a variety of ways, including psychological and physical effects.
  - Women with complete upper motor neuron injuries that affect the sacral spinal segments are unable to achieve psychogenic lubrication, while women with incomplete injuries often retain this capacity.
  - In addition to affecting lubrication, the level of spinal injury may affect the ability to reach orgasm and sexual desire.
- Sexual dysfunction has also been reported in women who have epilepsy, due to the side effects of the anti-epileptic drugs lamotrigine, gabapentin, and topiramate.

Menopause and Aging

- The effect of age on female sexual function is somewhat controversial. The National Health and Social Life Survey indicated that sexual problems may decrease with age, while the Prevalence of Female Sexual Problems Associated with Distress and Determinants of Treatment Seeking (PRESIDE) study, a survey completed by over 31,000 women, randomized to be a demographically representative sample of United States women and analyzed by Shifren and colleagues, found that sexual problems tend to increase with age.[6]
- Regardless, it is understood that menopause is associated with physiological and psychological changes that influence sexuality.
- The primary biological change that postmenopausal women experience is a decrease in circulating estrogen levels.

- Initially, estrogen deficiency accounts for irregular menstruation and diminished vaginal lubrication, leading to vaginal dryness, atrophy, and dyspareunia.
- Further estrogen loss is associated with changes in the muscular, vascular, and urogenital systems, as well as alterations in sleep, mood, and cognitive functioning that may directly and indirectly influence sexual function.

- Furthermore, the degree of impairment of sexual function may depend on whether the woman experiences surgical or natural menopause.
  - Natural menopause is associated with low estrogen, but ovarian androgen output continues to be maintained at premenopausal levels.
  - The PRESIDE study demonstrated that surgical, not natural, menopause was associated with orgasm difficulties. Additionally, the decrease in arousal experienced in postmenopausal women was determined to be greater in women after surgical menopause.
- On the other hand, hormonal changes alone may not account directly for changes in sexual function, as women of advanced age often simultaneously experience physical and psychosexual changes that may contribute to lower self-esteem and diminished sexual responsiveness and desire. Additionally, a woman's health status, medication use, changes in or dissatisfaction with her partner, and socioeconomic status may also affect sexuality.

Emotional and Psychiatric Factors

- Despite the presence or absence of organic disease, emotional and relational issues significantly affect sexual arousal in women.
- Female sexual function is greatly impacted by a woman's:
  - Relationship with her partner
  - Body image
  - Self-esteem
  - Ability to communicate her sexual needs
- In the Women's International Study of Health and Sexuality (WISHeS), emotional and psychological issues,

Library

College of Physicians & Surgeons of

300 - 669 Howe St.

as well as decrements in mental and physical health, were both independently associated with hypoactive sexual desire disorder.[7]

- Additionally, a history of sexual or physical abuse is a major risk factor for sexual problems, as was demonstrated by Lutfey and colleagues.[8] These researchers conducted an epidemiological study of over 3000 women to conclude that the odds of female sexual dysfunction were doubled when childhood or adult abuse had occurred.
- Psychiatric disorders are also strongly associated with female sexual dysfunction.
  - In the PRESIDE study, both depression and anxiety were significant correlates of distressing sexual problems.
- Also, medications used to treat depression can greatly affect the female sexual response cycle.
  - The most frequently used medications for uncomplicated depression are selective serotonin reuptake inhibitors, which often cause women to complain of decreased sexual desire, decreased sexual arousal, and decreased genital sensation with an associated difficulty in achieving orgasm.
  - Recently, however, Nurnberg et al. noticed that sildenafil can be successfully used to treat selective serotonin reuptake inhibitor–induced sexual dysfunction.[9]
- Antipsychotic medications are also associated with sexual dysfunction in both men and women.
  - The mechanism of action of these medications is inhibition of dopamine, which, as a side effect, causes an increase in prolactin, resulting in gonadal suppression.
  - Atypical (second generation) antipsychotic medications raise prolactin to a lesser degree than the typical antipsychotics, and thus may have less of an impact on sexual function.

Gynecologic Issues

- **Table 8.2** shows some of the gynecologic disorders that contribute to female sexual dysfunction.

Table 8.2   Gynecologic Etiologies of Female Sexual Dysfunction

• Dermatitis	• Painful bladder syndrome/ interstitial cystitis
• Vestibulitis	• Uterine fibroids
• Vulvar cancer	• Endometriosis
• Lichen sclerosis	• Myalgias
• Vaginismus	• Endometiral cancer
• Vaginal tissue atrophy	• Cervical cancer
• Vaginitis	• Clitoral adhesions
• Uterine prolapse	• Bartholin gland cysts
• Cystocele/rectocele	• Episiotomy scars
• Pelvic inflammatory disease	

- The etiology of female sexual dysfunction in the postpartum period is multifactorial.
  - In addition to anatomical and hormonal changes, the birth of an infant is associated with extraordinary fatigue and stress for the postpartum mother.
  - Nevertheless, Handa has indicated that within three months postpartum, 80–93% of women have resumed sexual intercourse.[10]
  - Sexual complaints, including dyspareunia and decreased desire, are common in the postpartum period and are expected to decrease with time.
    - Barett and associates demonstrated that 83% of primiparous women reported sexual difficulties at three months, and 64% at six months.[11]
  - However, due to the continued alterations in hormones, lactation may lead to a prolonged decrease in sexual activity, desire, and satisfaction.
- Pelvic floor or bladder dysfunction is an important cause of sexual dysfunction in women. In fact, as described in

the PRESIDE study, urinary incontinence is a significant correlate to distressing sexual problems.

- Salonia and colleagues determined that 26–47% of women with urinary incontinence report sexual dysfunction,[12] while Serati et al. stated that between 10 and 27% of women with urinary incontinence will experience leakage of urine during sexual intercourse, most often during penetration or orgasm.[13]
- Pelvic floor prolapse is also associated with female sexual complaints, and the rate of complaints is likely greater in those women who experience both prolapse and urinary incontinence.

■ Dyspareunia, or genital pain associated with sexual intercourse, may indicate a variety of underlying problems.

- In addition to being very prevalent in women with painful bladder syndrome/interstitial cystitis, dyspareunia is also a cardinal symptom of endometriosis.
- Furthermore, women with uterine fibroids may experience pain with intercourse, especially if the fibroids are located on the anterior surface or fundus of the uterus.

■ In addition to the above mentioned, there are many other gynecologic causes of female sexual dysfunction that contribute to physical, psychological, and sexual difficulties.

- Also, women who have undergone gynecologic surgeries, such as hysterectomies or excisions of vulvar malignancies, may experience feelings of decreased sexuality attributed to an alteration in or loss of psychological symbols of femininity.

Medications and Substance Effects on Female Sexual Dysfunction

■ Although often extensively researched in men, the effects of medications on sexual dysfunction in females are not as widely studied.

■ Conclusions about medications derived in the male population are frequently generalized to females.

- Often these conclusions are based on observation, as not all drug effects have been tested in randomized trials.

- Nevertheless, as described by Raina and associates, the most frequently cited agents that contribute to female sexual dysfunction include medications such as:
  - Anti-androgens
  - Antihypertensive agents
  - Drugs that act on the central nervous system, including antidepressants, anticonvulsants, and antipsychotics
  - Some recreational or illicit drugs[14]

Contraceptive Agents

- Contraceptive agents not only have profound effects on sexual behavior and beliefs, but may also elicit changes in sexual function.
- The two most widely used contraceptive medications are oral contraceptive pills (OCPs) and progestin-only agents.
  - OCPs act by suppression of pituitary lutenizing hormone secretion, which causes a decrease in ovarian testosterone levels. Also, the estrogen component of the pill increases sex hormone–binding globulin, resulting in a further decrease in free testosterone.
    - However, it remains unproven whether any effect on sexual function from OCP use is caused by the ensuing decrease in androgen activity.
      - Bancroft and colleagues showed that there is no correlation between inhibited sexual desire and testosterone levels.[15] These researchers treated OCP users who complained of decreased libido with exogenous androgens, and found no improvement of sexual function.
    - Furthermore, the decision to use OCPs is often associated with changes in sexual desire. Freedom from fear of unwanted pregnancy may enhance desire, while internal conflict over postponed pregnancy may lead to decreased desire.
    - Overall, there is little evidence that use of OCPs directly affect sexual desire or cause other sexual dysfunction.

- On the other hand, progestin-only agents may in fact have an effect on sexual function.
  - As determined by Matson and associates, depot medroxyprogesterone acetate may cause decreased libido in up to 15% of women, along with weight gain, depression, vaginal atrophy, and dyspareunia.[16]
  - Similarly, injectable progestins can lead to atrophic vaginitis and dyspareunia. However, these side effects can be easily alleviated with application of local estrogen cream.

Antihypertensive Medications

- Antihypertensives and cardiac drugs have been reported to affect sexual function by acting on the central or peripheral nervous system, the vascular system, or by having hormonal effects. These drugs include:
  - Adrenergic inhibiting agents
  - Diuretics
  - Vasodilators
  - Monoamine oxidase inhibitors
  - Anti-arrhythmics
  - Hypolipidemic agents
  - Digitalis
- Hanon and colleagues conducted a survey of over 450 patients treated for hypertension, and found that 49% of men and 18% of women reported sexual dysfunction.[17]
  - However, women who have hypertension commonly experience sexual dysfunction before treatment is initiated, often making it difficult to determine the true sexual side effect of the medication.
- Although sexual side effects of antihypertensive medication have been more extensively studied in men than women, adrenergic-inhibiting drugs are the most likely class of antihypertensives to elicit sexual complaints in both males and females.
  - Alpha-adrenergic agents such as clonidine have been reported to diminish desire, as well as to reduce subjective and physiological arousal in women, as

described by Meston and colleagues through use of a vaginal plethysmograph.[18]

- However, in general, there is still little known about the sexual effects of antihypertensive drugs in women.

Antidepressant Medications

- Sexual dysfunction is common in the general population, but is more common in those with depression.
- Many antidepressant medications are reported to affect sexual function, but controlling for pre-existing sexual dysfunction is difficult.
- Selective serotonin reuptake inhibitors, a commonly pre-scribed class of antidepressants, are reported to inhibit desire and impair orgasm in both men and women.
- In a cross-sectional patient survey of over 500 patients conducted by Williams and associates, 34% of men and approximately 33% of women were classified as experiencing antidepressant-induced sexual dysfunction.[19]
- Furthermore, Detke and colleagues determined that patients treated with the selective serotonin reuptake inhibitor paroxetine or serotonin-norepinephrine reuptake inhibitor duloxetine had a 62% and 46% incidence of acute treatment-emergent sexual dysfunction, respectively.[20] However, males and females were not differentiated in this study.
- Other antidepressant medications, such as bupropion, have been reported to have fewer sexual side effects than selective serotonin reuptake inhibitors.
  - In fact, Coleman et al. noted that more women treated with sertraline, a selective serotonin reuptake inhibitor, had orgasmic dysfunction than those treated with bupropion or a placebo.[21]

Antipsychotic Medications

- Similar to depression, sexual dysfunction is common in patients who have psychiatric disease, thus often making it difficult to distinguish the effects of the drug from the effects of the disease.

- Antipsychotics inhibit dopamine, resulting in an increase in serum prolactin, which can lead to a hypogonadal state and, in females, amenorrhea. A high serum prolactin is associated with inhibited sexual desire.
- Furthermore, atypical antipsychotic medications cause a greater increase in serum prolactin levels than typical antipsychotic agents, and are thus more likely to elicit sexual complaints in women, as well as in men.

Anti-epileptic Agents

- Sexual dysfunction is commonly reported in patients with epilepsy who are taking anti-epileptic medication such as lamotrigine, gabapentin, and topiramate.
- Of the three major anti-epileptic drugs, lamotigine is reported to cause the least change in sexual desire/frequency of desire in women, as described by Gil-Nagel and colleagues.[22]
- Grant and Oh, and Sun and associates, reported that gabapentin and topiramate, respectively, could induce orgasmic dysfunction in women.[23,24]

Illicit and Recreational Drugs

- In addition to prescription medications, illicit drugs and substance use may cause female sexual dysfunction.
- However, randomized, controlled trials of the effects of illicit drugs on sexual behavior are difficult to perform.
- Acute alcohol intoxication has been observed to affect sexual function by decreasing libido, interfering with arousal, and impeding orgasm in women.
- Chronic alcohol abuse in women leads to a hypogonadotropic state and resultant defeminization and loss of sexual function associated with dyspareunia and vaginal dryness.
- Similarly, Johnson, Phelps, and Cottler noted an association between marijuana use and dyspareunia and inhibited orgasm in an epidemiological study of over 3000 men and women that controlled for demographics, health, and psychiatric comorbidities.[25]

- The use of cocaine has been observed to cause sexual dysfunction in females via hyperprolactinism and decreased sexual desire.
  - Additionally, the use of cocaine is socially associated with sexual abuse, which often results in female sexual dysfunction.
- In men and women, the use of narcotics, especially methadone, is associated with decreased frequency of sexual contact and orgasm in women, as noted by Crowley and Simpson.[26]
- Nicotine may also inhibit physiological sexual arousal in women, as demonstrated by Harte and Meston in a randomized, double-blind, placebo-controlled crossover trial.[27]
- Furthermore, in addition to endocrine changes, substance abuse is frequently associated with relationship problems, poor physical and mental health, and financial burdens and lowered socioeconomic status, all of which may predispose a female to sexual dysfunction.

■ Conclusions

- Female sexual dysfunction is a highly prevalent, multidimensional problem with biological, psychological, and interpersonal determinants.
- The AFUD classification of FSD provides definitions and classifications that can assist clinicians with the diagnosis of these conditions.
- The effects of medications on FSD are not as widely studied, thus, conclusions about medication side effects on female sexual function are derived from what we know about male ED.
- Illicit drugs and substance abuse may cause FSD. This includes chronic alcohol abuse.

■ References

1.   The Global Study of Sexual Attitudes and Behaviors. *Int J Impot Res.* 2005;1:39–57.

2. Laumann E, Paik A, Rosen R. Sexual dysfunction in the United States: prevalence and predictors. *JAMA.* 1999;281:537–544.

3. Basson R, Berman J, Burnett A, et al. Report of the international consensus development conference on female sexual dysfunction: definitions and classifications. *J Urol.* 2000;163:888–893.

4. Park K, Goldstein I, Andry C, Siroky MB, Krane RJ, Azadzoi KM. Vasculogenic female sexual dysfunction: the hemodynamic basis for vaginal engorgement insufficiency and clitoral erectile insufficiency. *Int J Impot Res.* 1988;10:67.

5. Hutler BM, Lundberg PO. Sexual function in women with advanced multiple sclerosis. *J Neurol Neurosurg Psychiatry.* 1995;59:83–86.

6. Shifren JL, Monz BU, Russo PA, Segreti A, Johannes CB. Sexual problems and distress in United States women: prevalence and correlates. *Obstet Gynecol.* 2008;112:970–978.

7. Leiblum SR, Koochaki PE, Rodenberg CA, Barton IP, Rosen RC. Hypoactive sexual disorder in postmenopausal women: US results from the Women's International Study of Health and Sexuality (WISHeS). *Menopause.* 2006;13:46–56.

8. Lutfey KE, Link CL, Litman HJ, Rosen RC, McKinlay JB. An examination of the association of abuse (physical, sexual, or emotional) and female sexual dysfunction: results from the Boston Area Community Health Survey. *Fertil Steril.* 2008;90:957–964.

9. Nurnberg HG, Lauriello J, Hensley PL, Parker LM, Keith SJ. Sildenafil for iatrogenic seratonergic antidepressant medication-induced sexual dysfunction in 4 patients. *J Clin Psychiatry.* 1999;60:33–35.

10. Handa VL. Sexual function and childbirth. *Semin Perintol.* 2006;30:253–256.

11. Barett G, Pendry E, Peacock J, Victor C, Thakar R, Manyonda I. Women's sexual health after childbirth. *Brit J Obs Gynecol.* 2000;107:186–195.

12. Salonia A, Zanni G, Nappi RE, et al. Sexual dysfunction is common in women with lower urinary tract symptoms and urinary incontinence: results of a cross-sectional study. *Eur Urol.* 2004;45:642–648.

13. Serati M, Salvatore S, Uccella S, Nappi RE, Bolis P. Female urinary incontinence during intercourse: a review on an understudied problem for women's sexuality. *J Sex Med.* 2009;6:40–48.

14. Raina R, Pahlajani G, Kahn S, Gupta S, Agarwal A, Zippe CD. Female sexual dysfunction: classification, pathophysiology, and management. *Fertil Steril*. 2007;88: 1273–1284.

15. Bancroft J, Davidson DW, Warner P, Tyrer G. Androgens and sexual behaviour in women using oral contraceptives. *Clin Endocrinol*. 1980;12:327–340.

16. Matson SC, Henderson KA, McGrath GJ. Physical findings and symptoms of depot medroxyprogesterone acetate use in adolescent females. *J Pediatr Adolesc Gynecol*. 1997;10:18–23.

17. Hanon O, Mounier-Vehier C, Fauvel JP, et al. Sexual dysfunction in treated hypertensive patients. Results of a national survey. *Arch Mal Coeur Vaiss* 2002;95:673–677.

18. Meston CM, Gorzalka BB, Wright JM. Inhibition of subjective and physiological sexual arousal in women by clonidine. *Psychosom Med*. 1997;59:399–407.

19. Williams VS, Baldwin DS, Hogue SL, Fehnel SE, Hollis KA, Edin HM. Estimating the prevalence and impact of anti-depressant-induced sexual dysfunction in 2 European countries: a cross-sectional patient survey. *J Clin Psychiatry*. 2006;67:204–210.

20. Detke MJ, Wiltse CG, Mallinckrodt CH, McNamara RK, Demitrack MA, Bitter I. Duloxetine in the acute and long-term treatment of major depressive disorder: a placebo- and paroxetine-controlled trial. *Eur Neuropsychopharmacol*. 2004;14:457–470.

21. Coleman CC, Cunningham LA, Foster VJ, et al. Sexual dysfunction associated with the treatment of depression: a placebo-controlled comparison of bupropion sustained release and sertraline treatment. *Ann Clin Psychiatry*. 1999;11:205–215.

22. Gil-Nagel A, Lopez-Munoz F, Serratosa JM, Moncada I, Garcia-Garcia P, Alamo C. Effect of lamotrigine on sexual function in patients with epilepsy. *Seizure*. 2006;15:142–149.

23. Grant AC, Oh H. Gabapentin-induced anorgasmia in women. *Am J Psychiatry*. 2002;159:1247.

24. Sun C, Lay C, Broner S, Silberstein S, Tepper S, Newman L. Reversible anorgasmia with topiramate therapy for headache: a report of 7 patients. *Headache*. 2006;46:1450–1453.

25. Johnson SD, Phelps DL, Cottler LB. The association of sexual dysfunction and substance use among a community epidemiological sample. *Arch Sex Behav*. 2004;33:55–63.

26. Crowley TJ, Simpson R. Methadone dose and human sexual behavior. *Int J Addict*. 1978;13:285–295.
27. Harte CB, Meston CM. The inhibitory effects of nicotine on physiological sexual arousal in nonsmoking women: results from a randomized, double-blind, placebo-controlled, cross-over trial. *J Sex Med*. 2008;5:1184–1197.

CHAPTER 9

Physical Diagnosis and Testing

Chad P. Hubsher, MD ■ *Adam Luchey, MD* ■ *Stanley Zaslau, MD, MBA, FACS*

■ Introduction

- As previously discussed, female sexual dysfunction is a highly prevalent problem, with approximately 40% of women experiencing sexual complaints.
- However, few women volunteer a history of sexual dissatisfaction and, therefore, information needs to be actively elicited.
- Evaluation involves an open discussion with the patient, followed by a thorough physical exam and laboratory testing.
- Assessment of female sexual dysfunction can be used for both the purpose of diagnosis as well as measuring changes in specific parameters over time.
- Due to its multifactorial etiology, the ability to accurately and reliably assess sexual complaints in women is a difficult task for any health professional. A significant amount of time should be allocated for patient evaluation.

■ Patient History

- As female patients are unlikely to volunteer their history of sexual dysfunction to their medical providers, it is necessary to obtain a thorough medical history that includes medical, surgical, obstetric, gynecologic, psychiatric, and sexual information.

■ Medical History

- All concurrent medical disorders must be delineated.

- According to Sipski and colleagues, neurological diseases such as diabetes, multiple sclerosis, and spinal cord injuries can affect sexual function by impairing both arousal and orgasm.[1]
- Also, cardiovascular disease has been linked to female arousal disorder as a result of atherosclerosis of the vessels supplying the vagina and clitoris, as described by Berman and associates.[2]

Medications

- Several medications have been shown to impact libido, arousal, and orgasm. These include contraceptive agents, antihypertensive medications, antidepressive agents, antipsychotics, and anti-epileptic drugs.
- It is important to obtain a complete list of all medications the patient is taking as a simple switch of medication, for example from a selective serotonin reuptake inhibitor to a norepinephrine and dopamine reuptake inhibitor such as bupropion, may quickly alleviate the sexual complaints.

■ Surgical History

- Previous surgery that a patient has undergone, and the surgical details, may provide clues to the etiology of sexual dysfunction.
  - For example, a history of pelvic injury or trauma, as is seen with motor vehicle collisions, may be an important etiology for diminished sensation, or even pain.
- As described by Weber and colleagues,[3] certain surgical repairs, such as Burch bladder suspension with posterior colporrhaphy, may be associated with increased rates of dyspareunia postoperatively.
- Additionally, Vassallo and Karram have shown that vaginal stenosis may result from levatorplasty at the time of posterior colporrhaphy or aggressive trimming of the vaginal mucosa at the time of colporrhaphy, and, in turn, result in dyspareunia or apareunia.[4]
- Patients are often unaware of the exact procedure performed or details of their surgery, and thus medical records, such as an operative report, should be obtained

to gain further insight into the procedure and any complications that may have occurred during the surgery.

■ Obstetric and Gynecologic History

- Gynecologic conditions such as infections, endometriosis, fibroids, prolapse, and incontinence are common causes of female sexual dysfunction and should be addressed whenever possible.
- Additionally, it is important to discuss:
  - Menopausal status
  - Abnormal genital tract bleeding
  - Past episodes of urinary or fecal incontinence
  - Any incidence of vulvovaginal pruritis
  - Dryness, discharge, or pain
  - A complete pregnancy history
- Obstetric history, specifically detailing any previous cesarean or vaginal deliveries, including tears or episiotomy, may outline sites for potential denervation or dyspareunia.
- Additionally, removal of the ovaries may lead to sexual dysfunction secondary to estrogen or androgen depletion.

■ Psychiatric History

- It is imperative to discuss and explore any current or past psychiatric diseases, such as depression or anxiety, as these are part of the differential diagnosis of sexual dysfunction.
- Additionally, addiction disorders, including the use of cigarettes, alcohol, and/or illicit drugs, are important to discuss when discerning a cause of female sexual dysfunction.
- Finally, the patient should be screened for previous visits to a therapist. Although influential events in a patient's life, such as sexual assault or trauma, may not warrant a medical diagnosis, they still may serve as a potential contributor to sexual dysfunction.

■ Sexual History

- In addition to discussing basic gynecologic health, safe sex practices, and contraception, all women should be asked open-ended questions describing any sexual concerns they may have.

- If the patient indicates sexual concerns, then a comprehensive history should be obtained.
- At this time, the practitioner can ease patient anxiety by explaining that sexual history is part of a normal history and physical examination for all patients.
- It is important that assessment of sexual function take place in a private setting in which confidentiality is assured. It is imperative that the physician not make any assumptions, such as gender of sexual partner or that the patient's sexual behavior is limited to the identified partner or spouse.
- Patients rarely volunteer information concerning sexual dysfunction and, thus, it is key to identify the essential components of a sexual complaint.
  - **Table 9.1** lists questions devised by Basson that help to:
    - Elicit the patient's perception of the problem
    - Determine the problem's time line
    - Discern current health problems that might be affecting sexual function
    - Identify which components of the sexual response cycle may be compromised[5]
- Furthermore, sexuality questionnaires may delineate the source of the problem by asking questions that address libido, arousal, orgasm, pain, and relationship factors.

Sexuality Questionnaires

- Female sexual dysfunction diagnosis currently relies on a nonstandardized expert interview, as sexual function involves behaviors and psychological factors that are not amenable to direct observation.
- Two basic modes exist for the initial assessment of sexual function, clinician interviews and self-report through the use of questionnaires or diaries.
- Sexuality questionnaires play an integral role in the diagnosis and treatment of sexual dysfunction in today's office setting.

Table 9.1   Essential Questions to Include in a Sexual Assessment

- How does the patient describe the problem?

- How long has the problem been present?

- Was the onset sudden or gradual?

- Is the problem specific to a situation/partner or is it generalized?

- Were there likely precipitating events (biologic or situational)?

- Are there problems in the woman's primary sexual relationship (or any relationship in which the sexual problem is occurring)?

- Are there current life stressors that might be contributing to sexual problems?

- Is there guilt, depression, or anger that is not being directly acknowledged?

- Are there physical problems such as pain?

- Are there problems in desire, arousal, or orgasm?

- Is there a history of physical, emotional, or sexual abuse?

- Does the partner have any sexual problems?

Source: Adapted from Basson R. Taking the sexual history: part 1: eliciting the sexual concerns of your patient in primary care. *Med Aspects Hum Sex.* 2000;11:91–93.

- According to Althof and Symonds, they may be used to:
  - Identify/diagnose individuals with a particular dysfunction
  - Assess the severity of the dysfunction
  - Measure improvement of satisfaction with treatment
  - Examine the impact of the dysfunction on the individual's quality of life (e.g., relationship satisfaction, mood, sexual confidence)
  - Study the impact of the dysfunction on the partner and his or her quality of life[6]
- Since 1980, several brief assessment questionnaires that are specific to or inclusive of female sexual dysfunction

have been introduced and are suitable for office-based use, including:

  i. The Golombok Rust Inventory of Sexual Satisfaction (GRISS; 1987), created by Rust and Golombok, is a 28-item questionnaire that pertains to five domains specific to women, including vaginismus, anorgasmia, female avoidance, female nonsensuality, and female dissatisfaction.[7]

 ii. The Brief Index of Sexual Functioning for Women (BISF-W; 1994), created by Taylor, Rosen, and Leiblum, is a 22-item questionnaire that assesses female arousal, thoughts and desires, frequency of sexual activity, receptivity/initiation, pleasure/orgasm, relationship satisfaction, and problems that affect sexual function.[8] The index was subsequently revised by Mazer and colleagues to include a new scoring algorithm that provides composite scores and domain scores.[9]

iii. The Sexual Desire Inventory (SDI; 1996) is a 14-item questionnaire that was developed by Spector, Carey, and Steinberg.[10] Its intent is to measure dyadic sexual desire and solitary sexual desire.

 iv. The Derogatis Interview for Sexual Functioning (DISF/DISF-SRl; 1997) is a 25-item gender-keyed questionnaire that is suitable for both men and women.[11] It includes a total score as well as assesses five domains: cognition, arousal, behavior, orgasm, and drive or relationship.

  v. The Female Sexual Function Index (FSFI; 2000) is a 19-item questionnaire specific to women that was devised by Rosen and colleagues and is frequently used to evaluate female sexual dysfunction.[12] It comprises six domains: desire, subjective arousal, lubrication, orgasm, satisfaction, and pain.

 vi. The Menopausal Sexual Interest Questionnaire (MSIQ; 2004), developed by Rosen and associates, is a 10-item questionnaire that is specifically designed for use in menopausal women and contains three domains of sexual function: desire, responsiveness, and satisfaction.[13]

- In addition to providing information about the source of the sexual dysfunction, the results of sexuality questionnaires provide baseline scores that can be compared to later scores following intervention.
- Of the above-mentioned questionnaires, the Female Sexual Function Index (FSFI) (Appendix 1) is the most frequently used in office settings to evaluate female sexual dysfunction. The 19-item questionnaire is designed to measure sexual function over the past four weeks in each of the six aforementioned areas.
  - Since its development in 2000, the FSFI has undergone further psychometric tests that have confirmed its reliability and validity. One such test, performed by Meston, validated the FSFI in terms of the DSM-IV diagnoses of orgasmic disorder and hypoactive desire disorder.[14]
  - The FSFI is frequently used in clinical trials and is becoming the gold standard for the evaluation of women with sexual problems due to the fact that it is easy to use, relatively short, and considered reliable and valid.
  - A recent study by Wiegel and colleagues suggested that subjects scoring 26 or lower on the total FSFI score should be considered at risk for sexual dysfunction and should be further evaluated.[15]

■ Physical Examination

- Attention during the physical exam should be initially directed at the external genitalia, including the clitoris, labia, and vestibular glands.
  - Upon inspection, signs of atrophy or infection may be noted, in addition to episiotomy scars or previous surgical incision sites, which should be examined as they may be areas of tenderness on account of vaginal narrowing, scarring, or nerve entrapment.
- The pelvic floor should also be examined. The strength of the pelvic muscles can be graded based on degree of contraction during the pelvic examination.
  - Any evidence of prolapse (cystocele and/or rectocele) or disorders of the pelvic floor needs further evaluation.

- Additionally, neurological screening should be performed to assess sensation in the female genitalia.
- If the patient mentions or complains of pain, it is important to try to reproduce this complaint.
  - As described by Pauls, pain mapping may be achieved using a cotton swab on the vestibule.[16]
  - While the labia are held apart, the vestibule, vulva, hymen, and minor vestibular glands are touched gently with the swab.
  - Any elicited tenderness or erythema may suggest vulvar vestibulitis, which may require treatment.
- A digital internal examination should be performed to assess the levator muscles for spasms and pelvic organs for any masses or tenderness. Upon digital examination, the presence of vaginismus may also be noted as an involuntary contraction of the outer third of the vagina.

■ Laboratory Tests

- If hormonal deficiency is suspected, laboratory studies may be performed.
- Estradiol, follicle-stimulating hormone, and lutenizing hormone may be obtained if menopausal state is uncertain.
- Dehydroepiandrosterone, together with its sulfate ester (DHEA-S), may be measured to reflect adrenal androgen secretion, and can indicate an adrenal insufficiency.
- Thyroid-stimulating hormone may identify a thyroid dysfunction.
- Androgen production may be assessed by obtaining levels of total and free testosterone, total testosterone and sex hormone–binding globulin, or free testosterone and sex hormone–binding globulin.
  - As described by Guay, androgen measurements are highest in the morning and in the middle third of the menstrual cycle, approximately days 8 through 18, and, if possible, should be measured at this time.[17]
- In addition to the above-mentioned laboratory tests, a complete blood count, liver function tests, and lipid

profile may be helpful in managing the patients, especially if it is anticipated that medication may be used to treat the sexual dysfunction.

■ Special Tests

- Although useful for study purposes, specialized diagnostic testing such as duplex Doppler ultrasonography, vaginal pH measurements, and vaginal/clitoral sensory perception thresholds are not essential to evaluate and diagnose female patients with sexual dysfunction. Furthermore, these special tests are not widely available and often require expensive equipment.

■ Conclusions

- Medical professionals must actively question women who report sexual dysfunction, as this is a topic that is not often voluntarily discussed by the patient.
- Evaluation involves:
  - A discussion using open-ended questions to determine the patient's perception of the sexual problem
  - A detailed patient history, including medical, surgical, psychiatric, and obstetric and gynecologic histories
  - Administration of sexuality questionnaires to help delineate the source of the problem
  - A thorough physical exam and laboratory tests to assess the genitalia and measure the levels of various hormones in the blood, respectively.
- Upon completion of the evaluation, the patient should return for discussion to the physician's office without her partner.
- Using the American Foundation of Urologic Disease classification system, as described by Basson and colleagues at the international consensus development conference on female sexual dysfunction, the patient should be classified as falling into one or more categories, i.e., desire, arousal, orgasm, or pain disorders.[18]
  - It is important to ascertain the most distressing symptom, as patient complaints often overlap.

- Once the sexual complaints are classified and evaluated by the physician, therapeutic options can begin to be addressed.

■ References

1. Sipski ML, Alexander CJ, Rosen RC. Sexual response in women with spinal cord injuries: implications for our understanding of the able-bodied. *J Sex Marital Ther.* 1999;25:11–22.

2. Berman JB, Berman L, Goldstein I. Female sexual dysfunction: incidence, pathophysiology, evaluation and treatment options. *Urology.* 1999;54:385–391.

3. Weber AM, Walters MD, Piedmonte MR. Sexual function and vaginal anatomy in women before and after surgery for pelvic organ prolapse and urinary incontinence. *Am J Obstet Gynecol.* 2000;182:1610–1615.

4. Vassallo BJ, Karram MM. Management of iatrogenic vaginal constriction. *Obstet Gynecol.* 2003;101:512–520.

5. Basson R. Taking the sexual history: part 1: eliciting the sexual concerns of your patient in primary care. *Med Aspects Hum Sex.* 2000;11:91–95.

6. Althof SE, Symonds T. Patient reported outcomes used in the assessment of premature ejaculation. *Urol Clin North Am.* 2007;34:581–589.

7. Rust J, Golombok S. The GRISS: a psychometric instrument for the assessment of sexual dysfunction. *Arch Sex Behav.* 1986;15:157–165.

8. Taylor JF, Rosen RC, Leiblum SR. Self-report assessment of female sexual function: psychometric evaluation of the Brief Index for Sexual Functioning for Women. *Arch Sex Behav.* 1994;23:627–643.

9. Mazer NA, Leiblum SR, Rosen RC. The brief index of sexual functioning for women (BISF-W): a new scoring algorithm and comparison of normative and surgically menopausal populations. *Menopause.* 2000;7:350–363.

10. Spector IP, Carey MP, Steinberg L. The sexual desire inventory: development, factor structure, and evidence of reliability. *J Sex Marital Ther.* 1996;22:175–190.

11. Derogatis LR. The Derogatis Interview for Sexual Functioning (DISF/DISF-SR): an introductory report. *J Sex Marital Ther.* 1997;23:291–304.

12. Rosen R, Brown C, Heiman J, et al. The Female Sexual Function Index (FSFI): a multidimensional self-report instrument for the assessment of female sexual function. *J Sex Marital Ther.* 2000;26:191–208.

13. Rosen RC, Lobo RA, Block BA, Yang H-M, Zipfel LM. Menopausal Sexual Interest Questionnaire (MSIQ): a unidimensional scale for the assessment of sexual interest in postmenopausal women. *J Sex Marital Ther.* 2004;30(1):235–250.

14. Meston CM. Validation of the Female Sexual Function Index (FSFI) in women with female orgasmic disorder and in women with hypoactive sexual desire disorder. *J Sex Marital Ther.* 2003;29:39–46.

15. Wiegel M, Meston C, Rosen R. The Female Sexual Function Index (FSFI): cross-validation and development of clinical cutoff scores. *J Sex Marital Ther.* 2005;31:1–20.

16. Pauls RN, Kleeman SD, Karram MM. Female sexual dysfunction: principles of diagnosis and therapy. *Obstet Gynecol Surv.* 2005;60:196–205.

17. Guay AT. Screening for androgen deficiency in women: methodological and interpretative issues. *Fertil Steril.* 2002;77:S83–88.

18. Basson R, Berman J, Burnett A, et al. Report of the international consensus development conference on female sexual dysfunction: definitions and classifications. *J Urol.* 2000;163:888–893.

CHAPTER 10

Medical Therapies for Female Sexual Dysfunction

Chad P. Hubsher, MD ■ *Adam Luchey, MD* ■ *Stanley Zaslau, MD, MBA, FACS*

■ Introduction

- Treatment of female sexual dysfunction is complicated by the lack of a single causative agent, overlap of different types of dysfunction, and limited proven treatment options.
- Although sexual therapy and education, such as cognitive behavioral therapy, individual and couple therapy, and physiotherapy, continue to form the basis of treatment, there is limited research to demonstrate the benefit of psychotherapy.
- Recent developments in the treatment of male erectile dysfunction have led to the investigation of pharmacotherapy for sexual dysfunction in women.
- This chapter will attempt to describe the various noninvasive interventions to help ameliorate sexual dysfunction in women. However, prior to starting treatment, the patient should be evaluated thoroughly for all medical illnesses and drug history that may produce sexual dysfunction.

■ Psychotherapeutic Interventions

- Female sexual problems are generally the result of a complex interaction of biological and psychosocial factors.

- First-line treatment of female sexual dysfunction involves patient education and psychotherapeutic interventions that include:
  - Basic counseling
  - Cognitive behavioral therapy
  - Interventions for the individual woman
  - Couple therapy
- The goal of a psychotherapeutic treatment program is to assist the woman in both understanding her own physiology, feelings, and emotions and in communicating with her partner.

Basic Counseling and Education

- The initial treatment strategy of psychotherapeutic intervention, basic counseling, starts with the physician's readiness to give the patient time to talk about her sexuality and sexual problems.
- According to Annon, who developed a scheme for the behavioral treatment of sexual problems, inviting the patient to talk about her sexuality and entering into a dialogue with her physician may in itself provide a therapeutic effect, helping the patient not to feel so isolated and alone, but rather accepted and understood.[1]
  - As the patient tells her story, it is imperative that the physician engage in active listening. This means allowing her to tell the complete story and then summarizing the story back to her before asking specific questions.
- Many women have only partial knowledge of the basic facts of anatomy, physiology, and the human sexual response. Providing information about the differences between men and women, dispelling destructive myths concerning male and female sexuality, and educating the patient on the frequency and types of sexual problems women often experience can empower the patient by giving her knowledge and giving her problems a name.
  - As described by Bitzer and Brandenburg, some common myths that may be encountered include:
    - A healthy woman always has an orgasm.
    - Sex must lead to orgasm.

- Masturbation is only for singles.
- Not having sex leads to health problems.
- A man always wants sex and can always have it.
- Passion equals love.
- Sex must be spontaneous.
- Menopausal women lose interest in sex.
- Women want less sex than men.
- Women always need a lot of foreplay.
- Pornography is only for men (if at all).[2]

- Furthermore, patients should continue to educate themselves about their situation.
  - Women should be encouraged to read books or articles about sexual function and understand, for example, that not having orgasms during each sexual encounter does not mean that the experience was a failure and, as discussed by Walton and Thorton, clitoral stimulation may be more likely to lead to orgasm than coital intercourse.[2]
- Lifestyle changes are also an important aspect of education, as modification of known risk factors, including hypertension, hyperlipidemia, diabetes, cigarette smoking, or drug or alcohol abuse, is part of the treatment process. A healthy diet, adequate sleep, and exercise will promote physical and sexual well-being.

Cognitive Behavioral Therapy (CBT)

- In CBT, sexual dysfunction is looked upon as a learned behavior, either via classical conditioning, operant conditioning, or model learning.
- The result is a behavior sequence characterized by a specific sexual stimuli, response, and contingency.
- As described by Bitzer and Brandenburg, past experiences, resulting in sexual signals or bodily reactions, may lead to negative or positive emotional consequences that are stored in the amygdala and hippocampus.[3]
- CBT attempts to help people become aware of the stimuli, reaction, and consequence of sexual behavior, so that they may learn what enhances or inhibits their own sexual pleasure.

- Furthermore, patients are encouraged to understand their typical ways of thinking and the associated emotional or physical response, and to use CBT to help alter the resultant reaction.
  - For example, according to Bitzer and Brandenburg, the generic thought of lacking interest in sex may be accompanied by feelings of depression and frustration. This, in turn, could provoke reactions of defensiveness or wanting to fight, resulting in inhibition of the physical reactions of pleasure, such as vasodilation.[3]
  - CBT encourages changing the thought to lacking interest in sex intermittently and only in the usual way it is had. In this way, the patient may feel less depressed, which may lead to a better physical response.
- McCabe analyzed the effectiveness of a CBT program in 54 sexually dysfunctional females and demonstrated that after therapy, respondents experienced:
  - Lower levels of sexual dysfunction
  - More positive attitudes toward sex
  - Perceptions that sex was more enjoyable
  - Fewer affected aspects of sexual dysfunction in their relationship
  - Lower likelihood of perceiving themselves as a sexual failure[4]
- In fact, as discussed by Ghizzani, even when the etiology of female sexual dysfunction is organic, behavioral therapy may help patients change their behavior, overcome anger, sadness, and frustration, and communicate needs, and therefore improve their sexual function.[5]

Interventions Focusing on the Individual Female

- Psychotherapeutic interventions that focus on the individual woman attempt to help the patient become aware of her bodily signals and sexuality, while facilitating or inhibiting conditions related to pleasurable feelings.
- There are two types of therapeutic interventions that focus solely on the woman and have demonstrated some efficacy in improving female sexual dysfunction: pelvic floor and general body awareness exercises.

- According to Kegel, patients should become aware of the different elements of the pelvic floor, the movements of this part of the body, and the relationship between the pelvic floor muscles and their respiration.[6]
  - Physiotherapists and biofeedback instruments can promote this awareness, and women can learn to train their pelvic floor muscles and use them to increase proprioception of their vagina and vulva.
  - Exercises to increase pelvic floor awareness include:
    - Interrupting the flow of urine
    - Core exercises
    - Personal massage
    - Stretching
- General body awareness exercises, mainly described by LoPiccolo and Lobitz, encourage women to take an active role in their sexuality by exploring and experiencing their body.[7]
  - Each patient is encouraged to investigate her body by:
    - Observing her naked body in a mirror
    - Exploring her genitalia for sensitive areas and areas that can be stimulated
    - Progressively stimulating the genitalia, first by herself and then with a partner.
  - These exercises serve to reactivate the personal patterns of excitement, stimulation, and pleasure and help the patient find those postures and movements that lead to sexual excitement.
- A psychoanalytic, psychodynamic approach to the individual female, as described by Kaplan, views sexual problems as an internal conflict between sexual drive, originating in the id, and the societal norm, originating in the ideal self or superego.[8]
  - This creates a situation in which the bodily expression of the sexual drive, such as excitation and lubrication, is blocked, thus resulting in sexual dysfunction.
  - Psychodynamic-oriented therapy helps the patient overcome this internal conflict and encourages acceptance of the various elements of human sexuality, including fantasies and instincts.

Couple Therapy

- Sexual desire is often directed toward another person and, thus, sexual interaction becomes an issue of communication and exchange.
- Partners frequently have difficulty listening to each other and accepting the views, feelings, or thoughts of the other person.
- Partner counseling can teach basic listening skills, as well as the importance of respecting the partner and understanding how to express criticism without hurting the other.
- The goal is to improve communication and facilitate compromise.
- Masters and Johnson developed a basic form of couple sex therapy that combines behavioral, cognitive, and psychodynamic therapy.[9]
  - It involves home exercises combined with discussion topics in which the partners are helped to become aware of their thoughts and feelings during intimate interactions (**Table 10.1**).
  - The couple is then instructed to report back to the therapist to discuss any encountered difficulties or resistance to change and learn how to improve their communication.

■ Pharmacological Interventions

- There are a number of medications available for the treatment of female sexual dysfunction; however, no single therapy has been established as the gold standard.
- The study of sexual dysfunction in women has lagged behind research into male sexual health, resulting in slow progress in the development of pharmacological therapy for female sexual dysfunction.
- Nonetheless, estrogens, androgens, dopaminergic agents, nitric oxide donors, prostaglandins, and alpha-melanocyte-stimulating hormones are commonly used to treat female sexual dysfunction, although the results are variable.

Table 10.1   Couples Home Exercises and Discussion Topics

Exercises to Conduct at Home	Discussion and Reflection
Step 1: Caressing the body excluding the genitals, changing active and passive roles. Two times per week for 45 min.	What feels good, bad, irritating, or uncomfortable?
Step 2: Caressing the body including the genitals, changing active and passive roles. Two times per week for 45 min.	Exploring without the objective of stimulations, feelings, and communication about the experience. Feeling safe.
Step 3: Manual stimulation with changing roles and building up excitation.	How does it feel to play with stimulation, building it up and letting it subside?
Step 4: The man lies back and the woman sits on him, introducing the penis into the vagina.	The emotional significance of penetration, feeling close, and having the woman in control
Step 5: Movement and position experimentation	Sharing sexual stimulation with body movements and body expression

Estrogens

- For many years, estrogens have been the mainstay treatment of sexual dysfunction in women, and are currently the most commonly used medication for the treatment of female sexual dysfunction.
- Estrogen therapy is available in a variety of forms, including:
  - Oral tablets
  - Dermal patches
  - Vaginal pessaries
  - Vaginal estrogen tablets
  - Estrogen creams and jellies
- A meta-analysis conducted by Cardozo and associates revealed a strong correlation between levels of estrogen and sexual function in peri- and postmenopausal women.[10]

- Furthermore, irrespective of the route of administration, estrogen significantly improves dyspareunia and vaginal pH.

- Four randomized placebo-controlled studies by Casson et al., Nathorst-Boos et al., Sherwin, and Dennerstein et al. have all indicated that the improvement of sexual function observed with estrogen replacement in post-menopausal women was primarily based on local vaginal changes, such as relief of vaginal dryness, atrophy, and dyspareunia.[11–14]

- Although in postmenopausal women estrogen replacement therapy appears to improve sexual function, one must additionally consider the effects the estrogen has on serum testosterone.

  - In plasma, testosterone is largely bound to sex hormone–binding globulin, with only 1–2% of total circulating testosterone being free and biologically active.

  - The administration of estrogen replacement therapy increases production of sex hormone–binding globulin, which in turn may result in less available free testosterone and subsequently lead to a decrease in libido, as described by Sherwin.[15]

  - Therefore, it is plausible that postmenopausal women who have failed to correct their sexual dysfunction solely with estrogen replacement therapy may improve their sexual response by also being treated with testosterone. Estrogen replacement therapy is primarily indicated for vaginal dryness and dyspareunia, not decreased libido or frequency of sexual activity.

  - However, the systemic effects of estrogen replacement therapy are not observed with local estrogen therapy, such as patches, pessaries, creams, and jellies.

Androgens

- In clinical practice, testosterone is currently the most commonly used androgen, followed by dehydroepiandrosterone (DHEA) and androstenedione.

- Although there are no detailed guidelines, many clinicians believe that women with symptoms of low libido who have a total testosterone level less than 20 ng/dL and a free testosterone level of 0.9 or less may be prescribed testosterone substitution therapy.

- The prescribed dosages and duration of testosterone treatment vary on a case-by-case basis and, thus, routine monitoring is necessary.

- Adequacy of treatment is determined by the patient's self-assessment of improvement in sexual function; however, the side effects of weight gain, clitoromegaly, and increased facial hair should additionally be monitored.

- In females, the normal range of testosterone varies from 20 to 100 ng/dL.

- As a woman approaches menopause, she experiences a decline in ovarian function, a decrease in adrenal secretion, and an increase in peripheral androgen metabolism.
  - These changes result in a decrease in the levels of circulating androgens, such as DHEA, dehydroepiandrosterone sulfate (DHEA-S), androstenedione, and testosterone.

- According to Davis, women with testosterone deficiency tend to experience diminished sexual desire and fantasies, a decreased sense of vitality and well-being, and a loss of pubic hair.[16]

- A widely accepted indication for testosterone replacement therapy is female androgen deficiency syndrome.
  - In this disorder, women present with low libido, decreased motivation, fatigue, and a lack of well-being, but still show normal plasma estrogen levels and free serum testosterone levels in the lower third range.

- Similarly, hypoactive sexual desire disorder, the most common form of sexual dysfunction in women, may be treated with testosterone therapy, as determined by Laumann and colleagues.[17]

- Currently, only one form of testosterone, Estratest, which is a combination of estradiol and methyltestosterone and manufactured by Solvay Pharmaceuticals, has been approved in the United States for women with hypoactive sexual desire disorder.

- For the treatment to be effective, testosterone levels must be raised to the upper end of the normal range.
- According to several studies by Modelska and Milian, naturally and surgically menopausal women show greater improvement in psychological symptoms, such as lack of concentration, depression, and fatigue, as well as sexual function, including decreased libido, arousal, and inability to have an orgasm, when taking estrogen replacement therapy plus androgen therapy as compared to estrogen replacement therapy alone.[18]
- In women who have never had much sexual desire, or who have not experienced a change in libido, testosterone is probably not the appropriate therapy.
- However, as described by Burger and Davis, the addition of testosterone may be beneficial in women who have experienced a noticeable decline in desire and sexual function.[19]
- Therefore, it is important to properly assess a woman's sexual behavior and specific complaints of sexual dysfunction prior to deciding therapy regimens.

Oral Testosterone and DHEA

- Oral testosterone is rapidly metabolized by the liver and therefore has no bioavailability.
- The oral androgen testosterone undecanoate compounds in a lipid matrix to avoid degradation, but must be administered in substantial amounts two to three times a day to achieve clinical effects. Furthermore, this formulation is only approved for use in Europe and Canada.
- An orally active testosterone preparation available in the United States, known as methyltestosterone, works by reducing the androgen-binding capacity of sex hormone–binding globulin and, thus, elevates free and non-protein-bound testosterone.[20]
  - This facilitates endogenous and exogenous entry of androgens into the central nervous system and improves sexual function.
  - Methyltestosterone has been commonly used for treatment of decreased libido in postmenopausal women when it is combined with estradiol to form Estratest.

- Although methyltestosterone appears to improve decreased libido and ameliorate hypoactive sexual desire disorder, significant concerns, described by Simon, exist regarding possible liver toxicity.[21]
- The best way to deliver oral testosterone may be in the form of DHEA replacement.
  - In the United States, DHEA is currently available over the counter as a dietary supplement.
  - Guay and Jacobson have shown it to have positive effects on libido, and Hackbert and Heiman have shown it to have positive effects on sexual arousal, vaginal pulse amplitude, and vaginal blood flow.[22,23]
  - However, DHEA should be used with caution, as there is not enough research on dosages or duration for specific recommendations to be made.

Transdermal Testosterone

- Transdermal testosterone can be administered in the form of testosterone patches, creams, or gels and may achieve very high levels of testosterone with fewer side effects than oral testosterone.
- In a study by Shifren and colleagues, a testosterone patch increased frequency of sexual activity and pleasure/orgasm in women with bilateral oophorectomy who had impaired sexual function, despite estrogen replacement.[24]
- Alternatively, a testosterone cream, often between 1% and 3%, is available by prescription and may be applied to the clitoris and inner labia approximately half an hour before sexual activity to help improve sensation.
  - The applied testosterone cream helps to build up thin atrophic genital tissue, but constant use may result in enlargement of the clitoris or increased genital hair growth.
- Testosterone gels are also available in the United States and have the advantage of providing testosterone in a controlled-delivery format. However, as described by Redmond, these gels should be used with caution, as the relationship of testosterone gel dose to serum testosterone level has yet to be fully investigated.[25]

- An alternative method of delivery of testosterone is the subcutaneous administration of testosterone pellets, which are inserted in the abdominal wall every three to six months, often in conjunction with estradiol pellets.
  - The subcutaneous implantation of pellets containing testosterone and estradiol has been used in Great Britain and Australia, but is not common in the United States.
  - As described by Burger and associates, these hormonal implants provide significant improvement in libido, but may increase total testosterone to supraphysiological levels, causing side effects such as hirsutism and voice changes.[26]
- The route of administration, duration, and dosage of testosterone all influence the risk of androgen toxicity in women.
- It is important to find a balance that will help women with their libido without causing side effects of liver dysfunction or masculinization, including hirsutism, acne, deepening voice, weight gain, and alopecia.
- Hepatocellular damage is a serious side effect of testosterone replacement and liver function should be monitored whenever testosterone is administered.

Tibolone

- Tibolone is a synthetic steroid that has tissue-specific estrogenic, prostagenic, and androgenic properties that may improve sexual function, particularly sexual desire and arousal.
- The effects of tibolone, as described by Kloosterboer, have been attributed to the intrinsic capacity of the Δ4-isomer, a tissue metabolite of tibolone, which activates the androgen receptor, as well as to the reduction in sex hormone–binding globulin and the resulting increase in bioavailable testosterone.[27]
- Recent clinical trials by Egarter and colleagues and Baracat and associates reported beneficial effects of tibolone on sexual function in postmenopausal women, due to both an increase in genital blood flow and the central estrogenic/androgenic activity.[28,29]

- However, there is a need for future randomized and placebo-controlled trials in order to completely assess the effects of tibolone on sexual function and determine which subtypes of female sexual dysfunction may be effectively treated by tibolone compared to other available therapeutic options.
- At this time, tibolone has been approved for treatment of female sexual dysfunction only in Europe and Asia.

Sildenafil (Viagra)

- Sildenafil is an oral phosphodiesterase-5 (PDE-5) inhibitor, the introduction of which has revolutionized the treatment of erectile dysfunction in men. The mechanism of action in the penis is similar to that in the clitoris.
- PDE-5 inhibitors decrease the catabolism of guanosine monophosphate (cGMP), the second messenger in nitric oxide–mediated relaxation in clitoral and vaginal smooth muscles.
  - This results in an accumulation of cGMP in the clitoris.
  - Higher cGMP levels cause greater relaxation and dilation of the blood vessels, which may lead to greater and more prolonged clitoral engorgement.
- However, in 1999, Kaplan and colleagues reported no overall improvement in sexual function in postmenopausal women after sildenafil treatment, even though vaginal lubrication and clitoral sensitivity did increase.[30]
  - Similar results were observed in 2002 by Basson and associates, who conducted a large, randomized, controlled trial of women with female sexual arousal disorders and concluded that sildenafil did not improve sexual function.[31]
- Although the effectiveness of sildenafil has yet to be determined in the general population presenting with female sexual dysfunction, several investigators have reported it to increase sexual function in patients taking selective serotonin reuptake inhibitors (SSRIs).
  - In fact, Fava and associates and Shaller and colleagues determined that sildenafil improved several aspects of sexual function in women, especially in women whose

sexual dysfunction arises from the use of SSRI antide-pressants.[32,33] These areas in which improvement was seen include:

- Vaginal lubrication and clitoral sensitivity
- Arousal
- Frequency of sexual fantasies, sexual intercourse, and orgasm

- Sipski and colleagues have shown success with sildenafil in women with spinal cord injury (SCI). In her study of 19 women with SCI, significant increases in subjective arousal (SA) were observed with both sildenafil and sexual stimulation conditions. Maximal responses occurred when sildenafil was combined with visual and manual sexual stimulation.[34]

- However, at this time, sildenafil is not approved by the U.S. Food and Drug Administration (FDA) for treatment of female sexual dysfunction.

Vardenafil (Levitra) and Tadalafil (Cialis)

- Vardenafil and tadalafil are PDE-5 inhibitors, similar to sildenafil, that have been approved by the FDA for the treatment of erectile dysfunction in men.

- However, their role in the treatment of female sexual dysfunction has not been well studied, and the results of clinical studies remain inconclusive.

- There is some evidence that these medications may show promise, though. Angulo and colleagues conducted a study that showed that vardenafil increases clitoral and vaginal blood flow responses to pelvic nerve stimulation in female dogs.[35]

- At this time, none of the oral PDE-5 inhibitors, silde-nafil, vardenafil, or tadalafil, have been approved by the FDA for the treatment of female sexual dysfunction.

Phentolamine and Yohimbine

- Phentolamine and yohimbine are antagonists of the alpha-adrenergic receptor and in the past have been thought to be beneficial in treating sexual dysfunction in women.

- They are peripheral nonselective alpha-blockers that act by causing smooth muscle relaxation, resulting in vasodilatation.
- According to Rosen and colleagues, phentolamine has been shown to increase self-reported lubrication and sexual arousal.[36] Furthermore, it may be beneficial in estrogenized postmenopausal women with female sexual arousal disorder, as was determined by Rubio-Aurioles and associates.[37]
- Yohimbine, however, failed to show any improvement in placebo-controlled trials, including in patients with female sexual dysfunction induced by SSRIs, as determined by Michelson and colleagues.[38]
- Nonetheless, both phentolamine and yohimbine require further clinical evaluation to determine if and how they are effective in treating sexual dysfunction in women.

Other Medications

- To date, the results of clinical studies of a variety of drugs under evaluation for treatment of female sexual dysfunction have been inconclusive. These drugs include PDE-5 inhibitors (e.g., sildenafil, vardenafil, and tadalafil), peripheral nonselective alpha-blockers (e.g., phentolamine and yohimbine), vasoactive agents (e.g., apomorphine), L-arginine, oxytocin, prostaglandin E1, ginkgo biloba, caffeine, and low doses of psychostimulants.
- Currently, these medications are being tested in women with sexual dysfunction as single therapy or in combination with each other.

◼ Conclusions

- Sexual dysfunction in women is a multifactorial and complex problem that has only recently begun to be studied.
- Recent advances in anatomical, physiological, and psychological research have led to increased insight into female sexual function, suggesting that management of female sexual dysfunction should include both psychological and medical evaluation.

- Treatment of women with sexual problems often starts with sexual therapy and education.
  - However, spurred by the recent developments in treatment of male erectile dysfunction, the medical management of female sexual dysfunction is rapidly developing.
- Currently, hormonal options are the mainstay of treatment, especially in postmenopausal women. Still, there are a number of other medical therapies available that may play a role in future treatment options for women.
- Further studies are essential for creating effective treatment strategies and obtaining more insight into the pharmacotherapeutic similarities and differences between men and women.

■ References

1.   Annon J. The PLISSIT model: a proposed conceptual scheme for the behavioural treatment of sexual problems. *J Sex Educ Ther.* 1976;2:1–4.

2.   Walton B, Thorton T. Female sexual dysfunction. *Curr Women's Health Rep.* 2003;3:319–326.

3.   Bitzer J, Brandenburg U. Psychotherapeutic intervention for female sexual dysfunction. *Maturitas.* 2009;63:160–163.

4.   McCabe MP. Evaluation of a cognitive behavior therapy program for people with sexual dysfunction. *J Sex Marital Ther.* 2001;27:259–271.

5.   Ghizzani A, Razzi S, Fava A, Sartini A, Picucci K, Petraglia F. Management of sexual dysfunction in women. *J Endocrinol Invest.* 2003;26:137–138.

6.   Kegel AH. Sexual function in the pubococcygeus muscle. *West J Surg Obstet Gynecol.* 1952;60:521–524.

7.   LoPiccolo J, Lobitz WC. The role of masturbation in the treatment of orgasmic dysfunction. *Arch Sex Behav.* 1972;2:163–171.

8.   Kaplan HS. Editorial: Sex is psychosomatic. *J Sex Marital Ther.* 1975;1:275–276.

9.   Johnson VE, Masters WH. A team approach to the rapid diagnosis and treatment of sexual incompatibility. *Pac Med Surg.* 1964;72:371–375.

10. Cardozo L, Bachmann G, McClish D, Fonda D, Birgerson L. Meta-analysis of estrogen therapy in the management of

urogenital atrophy in postmenopausal women: second report of the Hormones and Urogenital Therapy Committee. *Obstet Gynecol.* 1998;92:722–727.

11. Casson PR, Elkind-Hirsch KE, Buster JE, Hornsby PJ, Carson SA, Snabes MC. Effect of postmenopausal estrogen replacement on circulating androgens. *Obstet Gynecol.* 1997;90:995–998.

12. Nathorst-Boos J, von Schoultz B, Carlstrom K. Elective ovarian removal and estrogen replacement therapy—effects on sexual life, psychological well-being and androgen status. *J Psychosom Obstet Gynaecol.* 1998;4:283–293.

13. Sherwin BB. The impact of different doses of estrogen and progestin on mood and sexual behavior in postmenopausal women. *J Clin Endocrinol Metab.* 1991;72:336–343.

14. Dennerstein L, Burrows GD, Wood C, Hyman G. Hormones and sexuality: effect of estrogen and progestogen. *Obstet Gynecol.* 1980;56:316–322.

15. Sherwin B. Use of combined estrogen-androgen preparations in the postmenopause: evidence from clinical studies. *Intl J Fertility Womens Med.* 1998;43:98–103.

16. Davis S. Testosterone deficiency in women. *J Reprod Med.* 2001;46:291–296.

17. Laumann EO, Paik A, Rosen RC. Sexual dysfunction in the United States: prevalence and predictors. *JAMA.* 1999;281:537–544.

18. Modelska K, Milian M. Treatment of female sexual dysfunction in postmenopausal women—what is the evidence? *Rev Gynaecol Pract.* 2004;4:121–124.

19. Burger H, Davis S. Should women be treated with testosterone? *Clin Endocrinol.* 1998;49:159–160.

20. Gooren LJ. A ten-year safety study of the oral androgen testosterone undecanoate. *J Androl.* 1994;15:212–215.

21. Simon JA. Safety of estrogen/androgen regimens. *J Reprod Med.* 2001;46:281–290.

22. Guay AT, Jacobson J. Decreased free testosterone and dehydroepiadosterone-sulfate (DHEA-S) levels in women with decreased libido. *J Sex Marital Ther.* 2002;28:129–142.

23. Hackbert L, Heiman JR. Acute dehydroepiandrosterone (DHEA) effects on sexual arousal in postmenopausal women. *J Womens Health Gend Based Med.* 2002;11:155–162.

24. Shifren JL, Braunstein GD, Simon JA, et al. Transdermal testosterone treatment in women with impaired sexual function after oophorectomy. *N Engl J Med.* 2000;343:682–688.

25. Redmond GP. Hormones and sexual function. *Int J Fertil Womens Med.* 1999;44:193–197.

26. Burger H, Hailes J, Nelson J, Menelaus M. Effect of combined implants of oestradiol and testosterone on libido in postmenopausal women. *Br Med J.* 1987;294:936–937.

27. Kloosterboer HJ. Tibolone: a steroid with tissue-specific mode of action. *J Steroid Biochem Mol Biol.* 2001;76:231–238.

28. Egarter C, Topcuoglu A, Vogl A, Sator M. Hormone replacement therapy with tibolone: effects on sexual functioning in postmenopausal women. *Acta Obstet Gynecol Scan.* 2002;81:649–653.

29. Baracat EC, Barbosa IC, Giordano MG, et al. A randomized open-label study of conjugated equine estrogens plus medroxyprogesterone acetate versus tibolone: effects on symptom control, bleeding pattern, lipid profile and tolerability. *Climacteric.* 2002;5:60–69.

30. Kaplan SA, Reis RB, Kohn IJ, et al. Safety and efficacy of sildenafil in postmenopausal women with sexual dysfunction. *Urology.* 1999;53:481–486.

31. Basson R, McInnes R, Smith MD, Hodgson G, Koppiker N. Efficacy and safety of sildenafil citrate in women with sexual dysfunction associated with female sexual arousal disorder. *J Womens Health Gend Based Med.* 2002;11:367–377.

32. Fava M, Rankin MA, Alpert JE, Nierenberg AA, Worthington JJ. An open trial of oral sildenafil in antidepressant-induced sexual dysfunction. *Psychother Psychosom.* 1998;67:328–331.

33. Shaller JL, Behar D. Sildenafil citrate for SSRI-induced sexual side effects. *Am J Psychiatry.* 1999;156:156–157.

34. Sipski ML, Rosen RC, Alexander CJ, Hamer RM. Sildenafil effects on sexual and cardiovascular responses in women with spinal cord injury. *Urology.* 2000;55:812–815.

35. Angulo J, Cuevas P, Cuevas B, Bischoff E, Saenz de Tejada I. Vardenafil enhances clitoral and vaginal blood flow responses to pelvic nerve stimulation in female dogs. *Int J Impot Res.* 2003;15:137–141.

36. Rosen RC, Phillips NA, Gendrano NC 3rd, Ferguson DM. Oral phentolamine and female sexual arousal disorder: a pilot study. *J Sex Marital Ther.* 1999;25:137–144.

37. Rubio-Aurioles E, Lopes M, Lipezker M, et al. Phentolamine mesylate in postmenopausal women with female sexual arousal disorder: a study. *J Sex Marital Ther* 2002;28:205–215.

38. Michelson D, Kociban K, Tamura R, Morrison MF. Mirtazapine, yohimbine or olanzapine augmentation therapy for serotonin reuptake associated female sexual dysfunction: a randomized, placebo controlled trial. *J Psychiatr Res.* 2002;36:147–152.

CHAPTER 11

Noninvasive Treatments for Female Sexual Dysfunction

Chad P. Hubsher, MD ■ *Aimee Rogers, MD* ■ *Stanley Zaslau, MD, MBA, FACS*

■ Introduction

- Noninvasive therapies encompass a wide range of modalities used to treat women with sexual problems.
- Due to the complex nature of female sexual dysfunction, each patient must be individually assessed to determine the best treatment methods to pursue.
- Examples of noninvasive therapy to treat sexual problems in women include:
  - Psychotherapeutic interventions and counseling
  - Lifestyle changes
  - Physical therapy that specifically addresses the pelvic anatomy and function, stimulation devices, sacral neuromodulation, and lubricants and moisturizers.
- Furthermore, it is often beneficial to the patient to be referred to a sex therapist or physical therapist who is specifically trained in educating and treating the patient in various noninvasive therapies.

■ Psychotherapeutic Interventions

- Female sexual problems are generally the result of a complex interaction of biological and psychosocial factors.
- First-line treatment of female sexual dysfunction involves patient education and psychotherapeutic interventions that include:
  - Basic counseling
  - Cognitive behavioral therapy

- • Interventions for the individual woman
- • Couple therapy
- ■ The goal of a psychotherapeutic treatment program is to assist the woman in understanding her own physiology, feelings, and emotions, and in communicating with her partner.

Basic Counseling and Education

- ■ The initial treatment strategy of psychotherapeutic intervention, basic counseling, starts with the physician's readiness to give the patient time to talk about her sexuality and sexual problems. This was previously described in Chapter 10.

Sex Therapy

- ■ Women with sexual dysfunction may additionally benefit from a referral to a sex therapist.
- ■ Sex therapists can educate a woman about the normal sexual response and effectively deal with cultural or religious concerns regarding sexuality.
- ■ Prior to referral, the clinician should reassure the patient that a therapist is a professional who deals with psychological issues regarding female sexual dysfunction, as there are many misconceptions about sex therapy. These range from sexual surrogacy to performing sexual acts in front of the therapist.
- ■ One of the most popular models used by sex therapists in treating female sexual dysfunction is the P-LI-SS-IT model, described by Annon in "Behavioral treatment of sexual problems: Brief therapy," which encompasses four levels of intervention.[1]
  - • The first level involves the practitioner creating a comfortable atmosphere, introducing the topic of sexuality, and giving permission (P) to discuss sexual concerns and enter into a dialogue with the clinician.
  - • The therapist then proceeds to address specific concerns, attempts to correct myths, and provides limited information (LI) about the human sexual response, differences between men and women, the frequency

of sexual problems, and the relationship of sexual problems with different life phases.

- The next level of intervention involves specific suggestions (SS), in which specific advice or treatment is given.
- For a majority of patients, these three steps should provide sufficient treatment; however, a small proportion of patients will need intensive therapy (IT) with frequent sessions of longer duration in order to improve their sexual complaints.
  - These patients' sexual dysfunction is often complicated by the coexistence of complex life issues, including psychiatric illnesses, interpersonal or intrapersonal conflict, or substance abuse.
- The sex therapist is trained to identify situations that require intensive therapy and make the appropriate medical referrals when deemed necessary.[2–4]

Cognitive Behavioral Therapy (CBT)

- In CBT, sexual dysfunction is looked upon as a learned behavior, either via classical conditioning, operant conditioning, or model learning.[5]
- The result is a behavior sequence characterized by a specific sexual stimuli, response, and contingency. This was discussed previously in Chapter 10.

Interventions Focusing on the Individual Female

- Therapeutic interventions that focus solely on the woman, such as a psychoanalytic approach or general body awareness exercises, have demonstrated some efficacy in improving female sexual dysfunction. This has been previously discussed in Chapter 10.

Couple Therapy

- Sexual desire is often directed toward another person and, thus, sexual interaction becomes an issue of communication and exchange. Partners frequently have difficulty listening to each other and accepting the views, feelings, or thoughts of the other person. Partner counseling can teach basic listening skills, as well as the importance of respecting the partner and understanding how to express criticism without hurting the other. This therapy was discussed in detail in Chapter 10.[6–8]

Lifestyle Changes

- Life events that cause an increase in fatigue or stress are frequently closely associated with sexual problems and a low libido.

- Reducing stress, either by applying better planning, organization, and time management skills or by attending stress-reducing activities, such as yoga or exercise classes, will likely improve sexual interest and satisfaction.

- Furthermore, getting help with child-care responsibilities and housework may also help to improve stress and daily fatigue, thereby improving sexual function.

- Also, encouraging couples to establish a regular "date night" that allows them to spend an occasional night away from family responsibilities may lead to significant improvements in sexual interest.

- In addition to minimizing stressful events and daily fatigue, there are a number of lifestyle changes that can be made to maximize one's potential for sexual satisfaction. Known risks factors of female sexual dysfunction include:
  - Hypertension
  - Hyperlipidemia
  - Diabetes
  - Cigarette smoking
  - Drug and alcohol abuse

- Reducing these risk factors and implementing a healthy diet, adequate nightly sleep, and daily exercise will promote physical and sexual well-being.

Pelvic Floor Rehabilitation

- Pelvic floor rehabilitation, a specialized field within the scope and practice of physical therapy, has clearly demonstrated effectiveness in the treatment of urinary and fecal incontinence.

- However, the pelvic floor is also a significant component of sexual function. It has been proposed that the pelvic floor muscles are active in female genital arousal and orgasm, and that hypotonus may be a significant component of sexual pain disorders in women.

- Additionally, conditions related to pelvic floor dysfunction, such as organ prolapse, lower urinary tract symptoms, and pelvic pain, are correlated with sexual dysfunction and therefore pelvic floor rehabilitation may aid in the treatment of female sexual dysfunction.

Role of Pelvic Floor in Female Sexual Function

- In addition to maintaining pelvic support and bowel and bladder continence, the muscles of the pelvic floor play an important role in female sexual function.

- For example, as described by Chambless and colleagues, a strong ischiocavernosus muscle that attaches to the clitoral hood is crucial for adequate genital arousal and attainment of orgasm in the female.[9,10]

- Additionally, Shafik proposed that during sexual activity, sexual pleasure is enhanced, for both the male and female, by contraction of the levator ani muscles.[11]

- Furthermore, Graber and associates explained that weak or deconditioned muscles may provide insufficient activity necessary for vaginal friction or blood flow, resulting in an inhibited orgasmic potential.[12]

- Also, syndromes that cause pelvic floor dysfunction and affect the urological system frequently have an effect on sexual function as well.
  - In fact, due to the relationship between urological and sexual problems, women with urinary problems should also be questioned about their sexual function.

- According to Handa and colleagues, women with urinary incontinence also reported low libido, vaginal dryness, painful intercourse, decreased orgasm rates and intensity, and decreased overall sexual satisfaction.[13]

- Similarly, Barber and associates determined that one-third of patients with prolapse reported that their pelvic floor condition affected their ability to have sexual relations.[14]

Pelvic Floor Hypotonus

- Pelvic floor muscle weakness has been reported as a source of urinary and sexual dysfunction.
- Often concomitant with pelvic floor hypotonus is a lack of sphincter control, which may lead to symptoms during intercourse of flatus and urinary or bowel leakage, and negatively impact sexual function.
- As described by Rosenbaum, in cases of prolapse of the posterior vaginal vault (rectocele), penile thrusting may put pressure on structures, causing bowel urgency and expelling of gas, and in more severe cases, fecal incontinence during sex.[15]
- According to Moran and associates, the pathophysiology leading to urinary incontinence during penetration may have to do with displacement of the anterior vaginal wall and bladder neck, or an increase in intra-abdominal pressure.[16]
  - It is thus reasonable to anticipate improvement with pelvic floor exercise.

Pelvic Floor Strengthening

- According to Kegel, patients should become aware of the different elements of the pelvic floor, the movements of this part of the body, and the relationship between it and their respiration.[17]
- Physiotherapists and biofeedback instruments can promote this awareness, and women can learn to train their pelvic floor muscles and to use them to increase proprioception of their vagina and vulva.
- Pelvic floor surface electromyography biofeedback involves insertion of a probe into the vagina, which measures the activity of the pelvic floor muscles, displaying them in graph form on a computer monitor.
  - The muscles can thus be visualized by the patient, who is given additional training to learn to relax, strengthen, stabilize, and coordinate them.
  - The goal of biofeedback is to normalize the pelvic floor muscle tone and improve contractile and resting stability.

- Exercises to increase pelvic floor awareness and strength include interrupting the flow of urine, core exercises, and personal massage.
- Additionally, as described by Mahoney, patients may be taught techniques to inhibit bladder contractions by using active pelvic floor contraction and providing reflex inhibition of the detrusor muscle via Mahoney's reflex.[18]

Mechanical Devices

- One nonpharmacological approach to the treatment of female sexual dysfunction is to use a mechanical device designed to increase blood flow to the clitoris and vagina.
- This device causes engorgement of the clitoris and a resultant improvement in:
  - Vaginal lubrication
  - Genital swelling and sensation
  - Orgasm
  - Overall sexual satisfaction
- There are two categories of mechanical devices that currently exist:
  - Mechanical vibrators
  - Clitoral vacuum engorgement devices

Mechanical Vibrators

- Mechanical vibrators have been used for decades to treat primary and secondary anorgasmia.
- Vibratory stimulation of the dorsal nerves in the clitoris induces clitoral engorgement, with consequent improvement of vaginal lubrication and enhancement of the female sexual response.
- However, vibratory stimulation may only be effective when these nerves are well vascularized. If the female sexual dysfunction is a result of diminished blood flow to the clitoris, labia, and vagina, stimulation with a mechanical vibrator may not achieve adequate engorgement because of poor blood flow to these diseased genital vessels.

Eros Clitoral Therapy Device

- The Eros Clitoral Therapy Device, the first FDA-approved nonpharmacological device for the treatment of female sexual dysfunction, is a battery-operated, hand-held apparatus that is placed over the clitoris to provide a gentle adjustable vacuum suction and a low-level vibratory sensation (Urometrics, Inc).

- The advantage of this device compared to a mechanical vibrator is that the vacuum suction allows engorgement of the clitoris even in the presence of diminished genital blood flow, as is seen with vascular disease.

- This device is designed to be used three or more times a week, for approximately five minutes at a time.

- Studies by Billups and colleagues and Wilson and associates both used patient questionnaires to show significant improvements in genital sensation, vaginal lubrication, orgasm, and sexual satisfaction after use of the Eros Clitoral Therapy Device in women with female sexual dysfunction.[19,20]

- Additionally, Munarriz and colleagues used duplex Doppler ultrasound to quantitatively measure clitoral blood flow before and after 10 minutes of stimulation with the Eros Clitoral Therapy Device.[21]
  - They determined that there was a significant increase in peak systolic velocity from 7.1 cm/sec to 26.2 cm/sec with use of the device in women with female sexual arousal disorder.
  - Similar significant increases were also observed in measurements of labial blood velocity.

- The Eros Clitoral Therapy Device provides an adequate alternative for patients who want to avoid use of pharmacological or hormonal agents for the treatment of female sexual dysfunction, particularly arousal and orgasm disorders.

Neuromodulation

- Over the past few years, neuromodulation has become an established treatment option for lower urinary tract symptoms.

- However, recently observations have been made of benefits beyond voiding disorders.
- This next section will describe various forms of neuromodulation and their effects on sexual function.

Sacral Neuromodulation (SNM)

- SNM is a relatively new therapy that is FDA-approved for the treatment of urinary urgency/frequency, urge incontinence, and nonobstructive urinary retention.
- The mechanism of action is largely unknown; however, it is thought to occur via alteration of the nerves that supply the bladder.
- Generally, a lead is implanted at the S3 foramen, while a pulse generator is placed permanently in a subcutaneous pocket over the buttocks.
- The pelvic, pudendal, and posterior femoral cutaneous nerves arise from S3, resulting in modulation of the motor innervation of the muscles of the perineum via the pudendal nerve and function of bowel and bladder via the pelvic nerve and its distal inferior hypogastric plexus.
- According to Bernstein and Peters, SNM may have added benefits, including:
  - Re-establishment of pelvic floor muscle awareness
  - Decrease in vestibulitis, vulvadynia, and bladder pain
  - Normalization of bowel function
  - Possible improvement of sexual dysfunction
- Little is known about the complex neural pathways that control female sexual function, but it has been hypothesized that SNM may have a direct impact on the female sexual response through the stimulation of the pelvic and pudendal nerves at the sacral roots, which are responsible for supplying the sensory innervation to the clitoris and pelvic musculature.
- However, at this time it is not definitively known whether the improvement of sexual function can be solely attributed to SNM, or possibly explained in part by the clinically significant enhancement of urinary symptoms.
- Additional studies examining the relationship between sacral and pudendal neuromodulation and sexual function

are needed to further evaluate the influence neuromodulation therapy has in women with sexual problems.

- These studies would optimally incorporate a large number of women who have sexual problems but no lower urinary tract dysfunction.

Transvaginal Electrical Stimulation (TES)

- TES is a conservative treatment option for urinary incontinence that was described over 45 years ago. It is used to stimulate nerve fibers and muscles by modifying the frequency of the conduction velocity of various nerve types.
- For example, at 5–10 Hz, TES affects the detrusor muscle by reflex inhibition with a pudendal to pelvic nerve reflex activation, and at 35–40 Hz, the pelvic floor muscles are stimulated through a pudendal nerve reflex loop.
  - As described by Berghmans and colleagues, randomized clinical trials involving TES advocate the use of 50 Hz for stress urinary incontinence and 10–20 Hz for urge urinary incontinence.[22]
- Recently, in addition to treating urinary incontinence, TES has been proposed in the treatment of female sexual dysfunction.
  - In a study by Giuseppe and colleagues, TES showed a significant improvement on urinary incontinence as well as sexual problems in women.[23]
  - Using questionnaires, it was noted that electrical stimulation significantly improved painful sexual disorders and orgasmic disorders, while also reducing the number of leakage incidents during intercourse.
  - However, these positive sexual function results correlated with a decrease in urinary dysfunction. Thus, at this time, the impact of TES on sexual function, independent of urinary incontinence, cannot be determined.

Percutaneous Tibial Nerve Stimulation (PTNS)

- PTNS has recently been introduced for managing lower urinary tract dysfunction.
- It was first described by McGuire and associates in 1983 and was based on the traditional Chinese practice of

using acupuncture points over the common peroneal or posterior tibial nerves to affect bladder activity.[24]

- However, details concerning its exact mechanism of action have yet to be elicited.

- Currently, this technique involves a 34-gauge needle inserted between the posterior margin of the tibia and soleus muscles, approximately 3–4 cm cephalad to the medial malleolus, and a stick-on electrode that is applied near the arch of the foot on the same leg.

- The needle and electrode are connected to a low-voltage Urosurge stimulator (Urosurge, Coralville, Iowa) that contains an adjustable pulse intensity of 0–10 mA, fixed pulse width of 200 μs, and a frequency of 20 Hz.

- Patients undergo weekly 30-minute treatment sessions for several weeks. If a benefit is perceived by the patient, often chronic maintenance treatment is continued.

- Similarly to TES, PTNS has also been recently proposed to treat female sexual dysfunction in addition to lower urinary tract dysfunction.
  - Van Balken conducted research using questionnaires to evaluate the effects of PTNS on sexual function in patients with lower urinary tract dysfunction.[25]
  - The study determined that sexual life, including overall satisfaction, libido, and frequency of sexual activities, were most likely to improve in women and patients with an overactive bladder undergoing PTNS therapy.
  - However, as with the previously described neuro-modulation techniques, further studies are needed to examine the effects PTNS has on sexual function, independent of lower urinary tract dysfunction.

Lubricants and Moisturizers

- During intercourse, lubricants and nonhormonal vaginal moisturizers can be useful in both pre- and postmenopausal women with vaginal dryness and dyspareunia.

- Although these agents may improve comfort during coitus and increase vaginal moisture, they do not reverse any atrophic vaginal changes that may be present.

- Water-soluble lubricants, such as K-Y Personal Lubricant and Astroglide, or silicone-based lubricants, including Eros and ID Millennium, are applied at the time of intercourse to decrease irritation.

- In contrast to lubricants that are applied at the time of coitus, Replens is a long-acting moisturizer that lasts up to three days and should be used on a regular schedule, being applied to the vaginal mucosa two to three times a week.

  - It works by binding to the vaginal epithelium, releasing purified water, and producing a moist film over the vaginal tissue.

  - In a randomized study by Bygdeman and Swahn comparing Replens to a vaginal estrogen preparation, dienoestrol, both agents significantly improved vaginal dryness, itching, irritation, and dyspareunia.[26]

  - Furthermore, when compared with each other, no difference was observed between the two agents Replens and dienoestrol.

■ Conclusions

- Sexual dysfunction in women is a complex process that can lend itself to many treatment options.

- Prior to beginning any treatment modality, it is important to thoroughly evaluate the patient and discuss with the patient the various options that may be pursued, including referring the patient to a physical or sex therapist.

- Furthermore, it is important for the patient to understand that when it comes to female sexual dysfunction, there is no quick-fix solution, and both the patient and the clinician must work together and be patient in order to obtain desirable results.

■ References

1. Annon J. The PLISSIT model: a proposed conceptual scheme for the behavioural treatment of sexual problems. *J Sex Educ Ther.* 1976;2:1–5.

2. Bitzer J, Brandenburg U. Psychotherapeutic intervention for female sexual dysfunction. *Maturitas.* 2009;63:160–163.

3. Walton B, Thorton T. Female sexual dysfunction. *Curr Women's Health Rep.* 2003;3:319–326.

4. Annon J.S. *Behavioral Treatment of Sexual Problems: Brief Therapy.* New York, NY: Harper & Row; 1976.

5. McCabe MP. Evaluation of a cognitive behavior therapy program for people with sexual dysfunction. *J Sex Marital Ther.* 2001;27:259–271.

6. Ghizzani A, Razi S, Fava A, Sartini A, Picucci K, Petraglia F. Management of sexual dysfunction in women. *J Endocrinol Invest.* 2003;26:137–138.

7. Kaplan HS. Editorial: Sex is psychosomatic. *J Sex Marital Ther.* 1975;1:275–276.

8. LoPiccolo J, Lobitz WC. The role of masturbation in the treatment of orgasmic dysfunction. *Arch Sex Behav.* 1972;2:163–171.

9. Johnson VE, Masters WH. A team approach to the rapid diagnosis and treatment of sexual incompatibility. *Pac Med Surg.* 1964;72:371–375.

10. Chambless DL, Sultan FE, Stern TE, O'Neill C, Garrison S, Jackson A. Effect of pubococcygeal exercise on coital orgasm in women. *J Consult Clin Psychol.* 984;52:114–118.

11. Shafik A. The role of the levator ani muscle in evacuation, sexual performance, and pelvic floor disorders. *Int Urogynecol J Pelvic Floor Dysfunct.* 2000;11:361–376.

12. Graber G, Kline-Graber G. Female orgasm: Role of the pubococcygeus muscle. *J Clin Psychiatry.* 1979;40:348–351.

13. Handa VL, Harvey L, Cundiff GW, Siddique SA, Kjerulff KH. Sexual function among women with urinary incontinence and pelvic organ prolapse. *Am J Obstet Gynecol.* 2004;191:751–756.

14. Barber MD, Visco AG, Wyman JF, Fantl JA, Bump RC. Sexual function in women with urinary incontinence and pelvic organ prolapse. *Obstet Gynecol.* 2002;99:281–289.

15. Rosenbaum TY. Pelvic floor involvement in male and female sexual dysfunction and the role of pelvic floor rehabilitation in treatment: a literature review. *J Sex Med.* 2007;4:4–13.

16. Moran PA, Dwyer PL, Ziccone SP. Urinary leakage during coitus in women. *J Obstet Gynaecol.* 1999;19:286–288.

17. Kegel AA. Sexual function in the pubococcygeus muscle. *West J Surg Obstet Gynecol.* 1952;60:521–525.

18. Mahoney DT. Integral storage and voiding reflexes: Neurophysiologic concept of continence and micturition. *Urology.* 1977;1:95–99.

19. Billups KL, Berman L, Berman J, Metz ME, Glennon ME, Goldstein I. A new non-pharmacological vacuum therapy for female sexual dysfunction. *J Sex Marital Ther.* 2001;27:435–441.

20. Wilson SK, Delk II JR, Billups KL. Treating symptoms of female sexual arousal disorder with the Eros clitoral therapy device. *J Gend Specif Med.* 2001;4:54–58.

21. Munarriz R, Maitland S, Garcia SP, Talakoub L, Goldstein I. A prospective Doppler ultrasonographic study in women with sexual arousal disorder to objectively assess genital engorgement following use of the EROS therapy. *J Sex Marital Ther.* 2003;29 supp l 1:85–94.

22. Berghmans LCM, Hendriks HJM, De Bie RA. Conservative treatment of urge urinary incontinence in women: a systematic review of randomized clinical trials. *Br J Urol.* 2000;85:254–263.

23. Giuseppe PG, Pace G, Vicentini C. Sexual function in women with urinary incontinence treated by pelvic floor transvaginal electrical stimulation. *J Sex Med.* 2007;4:702–706.

24. McGuire EJ, Zhang SC, Horwinski ER, Lytton B. Treatment of motor and sensory detrusor instability by electrical stimulation. *J Urol.* 1983;129:78–79.

25. Balken van MR, Verguns H, Bemelmans BLH. Sexual functioning in patients with lower urinary tract dysfunction improves after percutaneous tibial nerve stimulation. *Int J Impot Res.* 2006;18 (5):470–475.

26. Bygdeman M, Swahn ML. Replens versus dienoestrol cream in the symptomatic treatment of vaginal atrophy in postmenopausal women. *Maturitas.* 1996;23:259–263.

Female Sexual Function Index

Adapted from www.fsfiquestionnaire.com

Female Sexual Function Index (FSFI)

Subject Identifier _____ Date _____

INSTRUCTIONS: These questions ask about your sexual feelings and responses *during the past 4 weeks*. Please answer the following questions as honestly and clearly as possible. Your responses will be kept completely confidential. In answering these questions the following definitions apply:

Sexual activity can include caressing, foreplay, masturbation, and vaginal intercourse.

Sexual intercourse is defined as penile penetration (entry) of the vagina.

Sexual stimulation includes situations like foreplay with a partner, self-stimulation (masturbation), or sexual fantasy.

CHECK *ONLY* ONE BOX PER QUESTION.

Sexual desire or *interest* is a feeling that includes wanting to have a sexual experience, feeling receptive to a partner's sexual initiation, and thinking or fantasizing about having sex.

1. Over the past 4 weeks, how often did you feel sexual desire or interest?

   ☐ Almost always or always
   ☐ Most times (more than half the time)
   ☐ Sometimes (about half the time)
   ☐ A few times (less than half the time)
   ☐ Almost never or never

2. Over the past 4 weeks, how would you rate your level (degree) of sexual desire or interest?

- ☐ Very high
- ☐ High
- ☐ Moderate
- ☐ Low
- ☐ Very low or none at all

Sexual arousal is a feeling that includes both physical and mental aspects of sexual excitement. It may include feelings of warmth or tingling in the genitals, lubrication (wetness), or muscle contractions.

3. Over the past 4 weeks, how often did you feel sexually aroused ("turned on") during sexual activity or intercourse?

- ☐ No sexual activity
- ☐ Almost always or always
- ☐ Most times (more than half the time)
- ☐ Sometimes (about half the time)
- ☐ A few times (less than half the time)
- ☐ Almost never or never

4. Over the past 4 weeks, how would you rate your level of sexual arousal ("turn on") during sexual activity or intercourse?

- ☐ No sexual activity
- ☐ Very high
- ☐ High
- ☐ Moderate
- ☐ Low
- ☐ Very low or none at all

5. Over the past 4 weeks, how confident were you about becoming sexually aroused during sexual activity or intercourse?

- ☐ No sexual activity
- ☐ Very high confidence
- ☐ High confidence
- ☐ Moderate confidence
- ☐ Low confidence
- ☐ Very low or no confidence

6. Over the past 4 weeks, how often have you been satisfied with your arousal (excitement) during sexual activity or intercourse?

☐ No sexual activity
☐ Almost always or always
☐ Most times (more than half the time)
☐ Sometimes (about half the time)
☐ A few times (less than half the time)
☐ Almost never or never

7. Over the past 4 weeks, how often did you become lubricated ("wet") during sexual activity or intercourse?

☐ No sexual activity
☐ Almost always or always
☐ Most times (more than half the time)
☐ Sometimes (about half the time)
☐ A few times (less than half the time)
☐ Almost never or never

8. Over the past 4 weeks, how difficult was it to become lubricated ("wet") during sexual activity or intercourse?

☐ No sexual activity
☐ Extremely difficult or impossible
☐ Very difficult
☐ Difficult
☐ Slightly difficult
☐ Not difficult

9. Over the past 4 weeks, how often did you maintain your lubrication ("wetness") until completion of sexual activity or intercourse?

☐ No sexual activity
☐ Almost always or always
☐ Most times (more than half the time)
☐ Sometimes (about half the time)
☐ A few times (less than half the time)
☐ Almost never or never

10. Over the past 4 weeks, how difficult was it to maintain your lubrication ("wetness") until completion of sexual activity or intercourse?

☐ No sexual activity
☐ Extremely difficult or impossible
☐ Very difficult
☐ Difficult
☐ Slightly difficult
☐ Not difficult

11. Over the past 4 weeks, when you had sexual stimulation or intercourse, how often did you reach orgasm (climax)?

☐ No sexual activity
☐ Almost always or always
☐ Most times (more than half the time)
☐ Sometimes (about half the time)
☐ A few times (less than half the time)
☐ Almost never or never

12. Over the past 4 weeks, when you had sexual stimulation or intercourse, how difficult was it for you to reach orgasm (climax)?

☐ No sexual activity
☐ Extremely difficult or impossible
☐ Very difficult
☐ Difficult
☐ Slightly difficult
☐ Not difficult

13. Over the past 4 weeks, how satisfied were you with your ability to reach orgasm (climax) during sexual activity or intercourse?

☐ No sexual activity
☐ Very satisfied
☐ Moderately satisfied
☐ About equally satisfied and dissatisfied
☐ Moderately dissatisfied
☐ Very dissatisfied

14. Over the past 4 weeks, how satisfied have you been with the amount of emotional closeness during sexual activity between you and your partner?

☐ No sexual activity
☐ Very satisfied
☐ Moderately satisfied
☐ About equally satisfied and dissatisfied
☐ Moderately dissatisfied
☐ Very dissatisfied

15. Over the past 4 weeks, how satisfied have you been with your sexual relationship with your partner?

☐ Very satisfied
☐ Moderately satisfied
☐ About equally satisfied and dissatisfied
☐ Moderately dissatisfied
☐ Very dissatisfied

16. Over the past 4 weeks, how satisfied have you been with your overall sexual life?

☐ Very satisfied
☐ Moderately satisfied
☐ About equally satisfied and dissatisfied
☐ Moderately dissatisfied
☐ Very dissatisfied

17. Over the past 4 weeks, how often did you experience discomfort or pain *during* vaginal penetration?

☐ Did not attempt intercourse
☐ Almost always or always
☐ Most times (more than half the time)
☐ Sometimes (about half the time)
☐ A few times (less than half the time)
☐ Almost never or never

18. Over the past 4 weeks, how often did you experience discomfort or pain *following* vaginal penetration?

    ☐   Did not attempt intercourse
    ☐   Almost always or always
    ☐   Most times (more than half the time)
    ☐   Sometimes (about half the time)
    ☐   A few times (less than half the time)
    ☐   Almost never or never

19. Over the past 4 weeks, how would you rate your level (degree) of discomfort or pain during or following vaginal penetration?

    ☐   Did not attempt intercourse
    ☐   Very high
    ☐   High
    ☐   Moderate
    ☐   Low
    ☐   Very low or none at all

Thank you for completing this questionnaire
Copyright © 2000. All Rights Reserved.

Index

Library

College of Physicians and Surgeons of British Columbia

300-669 Howe Street Vancouver BC V6C 0B4